Collins *gem*

100 Ways to Boost Your Energy

D1079971

Theresa Cheung

First published in 2008 by Collins,
an imprint of HarperCollins Publishers Ltd
77–85 Fulham Palace Road
London
W6 8JB

www.collins.co.uk
Collins is a registered trademark of HarperCollins Publishers Ltd.

Text © HarperCollins Publishers 2008

8 7 6 5 4 3 2 1
12 11 10 09 08

A catalogue record for this book is available from the British Library.

ISBN 978-0-00-727588-5

Collins uses papers that are natural, renewable and recyclable
products made from wood grown in sustainable forests.
The manufacturing processes conform to the environmental
regulations of the country of origin.

Designed by Martin Brown
Printed and bound in China by Leo Paper

This is a general reference book and although care has been taken
to ensure the information is as up-to-date and accurate as possible,
it is no substitute for professional advice based on your personal
circumstances. Consult your doctor before making any major
changes to your diet. All recipes serve 1 unless otherwise stated.
Both metric and imperial measurements are given for the recipes,
use one set of measures only, not a mixture of both.

CONTENTS

....

INTRODUCTION

• •

TIRED ALL THE TIME?

Along with more time and more money, more energy is high on everyone's wish list. Without doubt, energy is an essential in today's overstretched, high-speed, 24/7 wired world; but it can be hard to recharge your batteries when there is a constant drain on your energy supplies.

Energy-shutdown is something most of us have experienced from time to time. Remember that drained feeling when, however much you have looked forward to a party, new movie or hot date, you just can't summon the energy to go? What is tougher to recognise, however, is low-key energy-drain. This is when you don't get that tired-all-over feeling but you do experience a gradual but increasing lack of enthusiasm for activities you used to get excited about. Getting out of bed in the morning seems harder, concentrating on what you are doing is a challenge and, most surprisingly, as you aren't normally like this, you find yourself getting worked up about the silliest things.

If this 'grumpy and run down' theme is starting to sound very familiar, don't despair. There are energy-drainers all around us – some obvious, some hidden. The good news is that you can find ways to deal with virtually all of them. Try one or all of the 100 simple and practical energy boosters in this book and, however hectic your lifestyle, you're bound to see your energy levels soar. Use them both as 'quick pick-me-ups' when the going gets tough, and as energisers to increase your stamina in the long run, so that you have all the get-up-and-go you need to rise and shine every day.

Use them to help put a spring in your step and a twinkle in your eyes so that you look and feel alert, vibrant and sparkling with energy.

PART ONE:

....

UNDERSTANDING ENERGY

What is energy?

....

Energy is life. It is the invisible force that animates the human body and permeates everything in the natural world, including animals, plants, trees and mountains, as well as the earth, sun, moon and stars. Whenever something moves, heats, cools, grows, changes or produces light or sound, energy is involved.

One of the simplest forms of energy is metabolic; this is the energy we get from the food we eat and the air we breathe. In short, energy means that birds can fly, winds can blow, the sun can shine, cars can go fast, light bulbs can glow and you can read this book. Without energy there would be nothing: no life, no movement, no light, no books ... nothing.

'Vital energy' is a term used to describe the collective physical energies of the mind and body working together to produce feelings of well-being. In other words, it means feeling glad to be alive, and bursting with health and energy. Typically children are bursting with vital energy – but an increasing number of adults are finding it harder and harder to remember the last time they felt like that.

Energy and health

A healthy person is a person who has a sense of well-being characterised by a high level of energy and the ability to cope with stress. Feeling tired and stressed a lot of the time is not healthy. Unfortunately, many of us unconsciously settle for energy levels that are lacklustre, in the belief that it is normal to 'run on empty'. But low energy levels are certainly not normal or healthy.

Energy is our most precious human resource. If we don't have it, not only is our immunity low and our health at risk, but we don't have the 'oomph' we need to rise to the challenge of work, have fulfilling relationships and experience the joy of being alive that is our birthright. If we don't have energy, we are simply going through the motions of life.

Although energy can put a spring in our step and help keep disease at bay, it's important to remember that healthy energy levels are also *balanced* energy levels. In other words, we need to have the energy to meet the challenges of life without going into overdrive. Overdrive is certainly not good for our health and well-being because it makes it hard to switch off and relax, and increases our risk of stress and poor health. What we need to be aiming for isn't constantly high energy levels but a steady flow of balanced physical, emotional and mental energy; these balanced levels are essential if we are genuinely to experience good health and vitality.

Energy peaks and troughs

It's important to know that our energy level won't remain constant throughout the day; there will be natural dips. In fact, scientists have identified 2.16 p.m. as the time most of us experience an energy dip, so if you get a slump around this time it does not mean that anything is 'wrong'.

Some energy lows are of our own doing – caused by those late nights or too much caffeine – but the conductor of our energy levels is a cluster of cells that lie deep within our brains, directing our daily release of hormones, our shifts in body temperature and our blood pressure. This conductor produces what are called 'circadian rhythms'.

Research has shown that one of the most powerful regulators of our internal body clock or circadian rhythm is *light*. When photoreceptors in our eyes and other places absorb light, they send a signal to our brains to stop producing melatonin, the so-called sleep hormone. With light comes a cessation of melatonin production, and our gradually increasing body temperature makes us feel alert. During the day our temperature fluctuates, rising in the mid-morning, hitting a low at around 3 p.m. and then rising again in mid-afternoon; this could explain why we often get a second wind around this time. By 11 p.m., when the lights are usually turned off, melatonin production starts and temperature, heart rate and blood pressure drop in preparation for sleep.

It's important to understand the physical rhythms that guide our days so we can learn to make the most of energy peaks and prepare ourselves for energy troughs. One way to keep track is to have an energy diary and write down the times when you feel alert or tired during the day. Once you are aware of your 'downtime', you can plan your life accordingly. For example, if you get a slump at around 3 p.m. you can avoid planning meetings at that time – or use some of the instant pick-me-up tips on pages 175–89. If, however, you find that your energy is constantly low or that you have more troughs than peaks during the day, your energy levels are lower than they should be.

Symtoms of low energy

Symptoms of low energy vary from person to person. In general when your energy is low, although you may be able to cope with your normal routine, you've lost that spring in your step and anything that requires a little more effort tires you quickly. You may often simply wake up tired and just have a general feeling of being out of sorts.

To rate your energy levels, answer the following questions:

☐ When you wake up in the morning, do you drag yourself reluctantly out of bed?

☐ Do you find yourself longing for an afternoon nap in the morning?

☐ At the end of the day, is slumping in front of the TV all that you want to do?

☐ During meetings do you easily become distracted or bored, or find it hard to keep your eyes open?

☐ Do you sometimes feel that you haven't got the energy to get through the day?

☐ Do you fall asleep the moment your head hits the pillow?

☐ Do you often feel so wound up that it is hard to get to sleep?

☐ Does seeing or talking to friends seem like a huge effort sometimes?

☐ Is it hard to remember things or to concentrate at work?

☐ Do you find yourself getting worked up or impatient about the smallest things?

❑ Do you need caffeine or other stimulants to help you through the day?

❑ Are you susceptible to colds and other minor illnesses?

❑ Do you find it difficult to raise much enthusiasm for doing anything at all?

❑ Is it hard for you to accept or deal with change?

❑ Has it been a few weeks since you had a good laugh?

If you have ticked more than two boxes, this suggests that your energy levels are lower than they should be.

The causes of low energy: energy-drainers

Low energy is a concept that's hard to define. Everyone will have their own idea of what being tired means, and we all feel tired once in a while; but if you feel that you have lost some of your zest for life, your energy levels are lower than they should be and you need to find out why.

Identifying what is causing your energy to dip is important because once you know what is robbing you of your vitality, you can then take steps to avoid it or manage it positively.

In most cases there is not one single cause that contributes to low energy, but a combination of several factors. Listed below are some of the most common energy-drainers including poor-quality sleep, unhealthy eating, lack of exercise, environmental factors, stress and underlying medical conditions. Review the information and use it to help you recognise your most common energy-drainers so that you can make positive changes to your diet and/or lifestyle, or seek medical advice. Then you are all set to re-energise yourself by cultivating the energy-boosting advice from page 41 onwards.

Sleep deprivation

Not getting a good night's sleep is a common reason for low energy during the day. Between 7 and 8 hours of quality sleep a night is what most people need. Anything less than that and your immune system and your body's battery-boosting systems suffer. This can lead to poor concentration, erratic judgement, slow reaction times, memory problems and poor physical performance, as well as mood swings and irritability.

Your sleep–waking cycle is regulated by the stimulus of sunrise and sunset, but a frantic and unhealthy lifestyle can upset your body clock, causing sleeping problems, fatigue and chronic sleep deprivation. It is certainly possible to train yourself to get by on less sleep, but during sleep both body and brain are restored, rejuvenated and re-energized. So why would you skimp on such a valuable energy-boosting resource? To find out if you are getting enough quality sleep, do any of the following apply to you?

- Needing an alarm clock to wake up.
- Falling asleep within 5 minutes of getting into bed.
- Trouble getting out of bed in the mornings.
- Drowsiness during the day and especially around 4 p.m..
- Dozing off while watching TV, after a heavy lunch, or in a public place such as a meeting or at work.
- Excessive yawning.
- Need for caffeine and stimulants to get through the day.

If two or more items on this list apply to you, this suggests a lack of good-quality sleep. You should pay particular attention to the good sleep advice on pages 42–56.

Unhealthy diet

A well-balanced, healthy diet is essential for high energy levels. At its most basic level, what you eat and drink is the fuel that your body and brain need to function at their peak. Skimp on the quality of that fuel and you will pay the price with weight gain and low energy. Skipping breakfast, not drinking enough water, over-eating, dieting, eating on the run, consumption of caffeine and alcohol and eating a lot of refined, processed foods are the major causes of low energy levels.

Rate your diet

- Do you eat breakfast every morning?
- Do you eat at least 2,000 calories each day, mostly comprised of healthy, freshly prepared whole foods?
- Do you grab a piece of fruit and a handful of nuts and seeds instead of a bar of chocolate to fight your midday doldrums?
- Do you limit yourself to fewer than three cups of coffee every day?
- Do you drink six to eight glasses of fluid every day (colas and coffee don't count!)?
- Do you make sure you eat something every couple of hours?
- Do you sit down and take your time when you have a meal, chewing your food thoroughly?

More than one 'no' answer suggests that your diet may play a role in your energy crisis. You should therefore pay particular attention to the diet-related energy-boosting tips on pages 57–91.

The sugar blues

Almost all of your energy comes from glucose (sugar). Therefore, maintaining an even blood sugar level is essential to ensure your energy levels are healthy and your mood upbeat. The best way to control your blood sugar levels is to watch what you eat, in particular what carbohydrates you eat.

Carbohydrates are broken down into sugar, which gives your body energy. The speed at which this process occurs affects your mood, weight and energy, and your ability to cope with stress. Some carbohydrates raise your blood sugar levels quickly, while others take their time. Fast-releasing carbohydrates, such as sugar and white flour, send your blood sugar levels rocketing very quickly after eating them, so you get a burst of energy. Unfortunately this is soon followed by a rapid dip in sugar which means you feel tired and sleepy – that 'energy trough' –

and you crave another fix all over again. Slow-releasing carbohydrates, on the other hand, such as wholegrains and vegetables, give you a steady release of sugar and energy, keeping your energy levels constant.

Eating food that is going to keep your blood sugar levels and your energy levels constant is therefore vital. The rate at which food releases glucose into your bloodstream can be measured on the glycaemic index (GI). If you haven't got the time to work with the GI, a general rule is that the more natural and unprocessed a food is, the lower it is on the GI and the better it is for you. In a nutshell, the closer food is to its natural, unrefined state, the richer it is in nutrients and the greater its energy potential. A diet that is rich in fresh, natural wholegrains, fruits and vegetables, legumes, nuts and seeds, and low in red meat, sugar, white flour, refined and processed foods which have been stripped of their fibre, vitamin and mineral energy, fast foods and ready meals, will help you avoid the dips in energy and mood that come with fluctuating blood sugar levels.

For more advice on energy-boosting nutrients and foods, check out the tips on pages 84–5.

Stimulants

When blood sugar levels dip or fatigue sets in, many people turn to stimulants such as tea, coffee, sugary drinks, cigarettes and chocolate to keep them going. Although they can give you a temporary high, the long-term effects of stimulants are always bad.

Alcohol is made from yeast and has a similar effect to sugar in your body, giving you a temporary high followed by a long low.

Coffee is a diuretic which depletes your body of nutrients and it also contains caffeine which disturbs normal sleep patterns.

Many **fizzy drinks** contain caffeine, as well as sugar and colourings which act as stimulants.

Tea is a stimulant with similar but weaker effects to coffee, and it contains tannin which interferes with the absorption of minerals.

Chocolate contains theobromine which has an action similar to, but not as strong as, caffeine.

Medications for the relief of headaches also contain caffeine.

Cigarettes contain cancerous chemicals and the stimulant nicotine which is sedative in large amounts.

Stimulants are your body's greatest energy-drainers, so one of the most important steps you can take to beat fatigue is to give up or cut down on stimulants. Giving up all these stimulants at once would be impossible for most people, as well as being incredibly stressful. The first step, therefore, is to identify which stimulants you are using as pick-me-ups to get you going when your energy is flagging, and to cut consumption of them down gradually.

To cut down on stimulants without suffering try the following:

Sugar: When you crave something sweet, eat some fruit. Don't replace sugar with sugar substitutes, as these do not help you re-educate your taste buds. Take the sugar bowl off the table and give yourself a month to gradually cut down. Read labels and find healthier alternatives. Stick with it and after a few weeks you will find that your taste buds adapt.

Coffee: Coffee is addictive and it takes about a week to break the habit. You may find yourself feeling groggy for a few days, but this will remind you how addictive and bad for you too much coffee is. Instead of coffee, drink herbal teas or coffee alternatives such as dandelion coffee. After a week you can go back to one or two cups of coffee a day, but as a treat, not as an energy booster.

Tea: Tea isn't as energy-draining as coffee unless you drink gallons of it a day. Two or three cups a day is fine, but it is still worth experimenting with herbal teas or drinking your tea slightly weaker.

Chocolate: If you adore chocolate, you don't need to give it up completely. Just eat it in moderation, for example four times a week rather than every day. Most important of all, don't use it as a pick-me-up as it will have the opposite effect. Go for fruit with a handful of nuts and seeds instead if you need something sweet and satisfying.

Alcohol: If you drink a lot, start by reminding yourself that you don't actually need to have a glass in your hand to have a good time. Set yourself a weekly target of five to seven drinks a week and stick to it. If you find this impossible, seek professional advice.

Smoking: This is perhaps one of the hardest energy-draining habits to break and one for which you may need to seek the advice of your doctor if you want to quit. It really is worth persisting, though, as many people who give up find that their energy levels soar. To reduce your cravings you need to boost your body's ability to eliminate chemicals. A healthy diet, plenty of exercise and drinking lots of water can all help detoxify your body.

Dieting

If you're cutting calories and skipping meals in an effort to control your weight, there's a good chance you're simply not giving your body the essential nutritional building-blocks it needs to operate at peak capacity.

Dieting or going for long periods without food is the worst thing you can do for your energy levels. Not only will nutritional deficiencies trigger fatigue, your blood sugar levels will plummet and, as mentioned previously, low blood sugar levels are directly related to fatigue. Eating regularly scheduled meals, with healthy snacks in between, will ensure that your blood sugar levels are balanced and you have the necessary fuel to perform at your best all day.

When you skip meals you fail to replenish your energy reserves, so always have breakfast, aim for a good lunch during the day, and keep nutritious snacks to hand. Avoid big meals because they divert blood flow to your digestive tract, making you feel heavy and tired. It is vital that you avoid large meals at bedtime, as your body will spend the night processing food rather than healing and repairing tissue. Eat little and often (be a 'grazer' not a 'gorger'), and have a little healthy protein with each meal or snack – such as some nuts with a piece of fruit – because protein has a stabilizing effect on your blood sugar.

You would not expect your car to run on empty, so treat yourself as well as your car. You'll know that driving at a constant speed gives your car the best mileage. Likewise, if you keep yourself well fed throughout the day, your metabolism will be at its best too, which means you have more energy and are in calorie-burning mode.

Sedentary lifestyle
A lifestyle that is inactive or sedentary can have a negative affect on your digestive system and reduce your respiratory capacity, place strain on your heart and cardiovascular system, and cause loss of muscle mass and stamina. On top of all

that, a sedentary lifestyle can dull your powers of concentration, and if you spend too much time indoors you won't be getting the oxygen energising benefits of fresh air.

To find out if your lifestyle is too sedentary, answer the following questions:

- Is your life so busy that you haven't got time to exercise?
- Is your favourite hobby channel-surfing from the couch?
- Do you circle the parking lot for 5 minutes instead of parking in the first spot you see and taking a 5-minute walk?
- Do you spend most of the day at your desk or indoors?
- When you sit down do you slump almost immediately?

If there is more than one 'yes' answer, your lifestyle may be the cause of your energy roller-coaster and you should pay special attention to the boosting energy with exercise tips on pages 92–109.

Toxic environment

Your body creates energy not just from nutrients but from oxygen and even positive emotions; therefore your energy levels will be affected by the space around you and the state of mind you are in. The room you work in, the energy in your home, the environment outside your office or house – all these have an effect on the way you feel and the amount of energy you expend in keeping going. For example, if you are constantly exposed to packed streets, buses, trains, car fumes, busy shops, clutter and lack of natural light and greenery, your body and mind are being bombarded with energy-draining stimuli. On the other hand, nature, in particular green leafy forests, clean air and surroundings that are calm and uplifting, can re-energise you.

Hidden energy-zappers such as pollution, additives, preservatives, environmental toxins, watching too much TV (which can suppress production of the sleep hormone) and excessive use of mobile phones and computers, can all drain your energy. Lack of fresh air by staying too long indoors and depriving yourself of energising oxygen is another contributing factor.

If you think that the environment you live and work in may be draining your resources, pay attention to the energy tips on pages 110–43.

Stress

Stress is a major cause of low energy and can affect you mentally, physically and emotionally. It's well known that many illnesses are stress related, including digestive disorders such as irritable bowel syndrome, respiratory problems such as asthma, high blood pressure and tension headaches.

Heavy workloads or trying to fit in as many tasks as possible can cause a great deal of stress. Many people are constantly working against the clock and this can slowly sap energy and enthusiasm, resulting in dependency on stimulants such as caffeine to get you through the day and alcohol to help you unwind at night. The benefits of these are fleeting and the adverse effects are long term. Juggling the needs of family and work can crank up the pressure, as can financial worries, relationship problems, feeling lonely and other personal problems that drag you down.

If you do feel that you are more anxious and stressed than you should be and that this is making you feel drained and tired, pay particular attention to the energy tips on pages 171–74.

Boredom

Too much stress will drain your energy, but what is often overlooked is that a certain amount of stress is essential for a healthy, happy life. In moderation, stress sharpens your reflexes, heightens your responses and gives you the energy to cope with demanding and difficult situations. If your life were totally stress-free you wouldn't have challenges. Life would be predictable. You wouldn't have to adjust to change. You wouldn't ever feel pressured. You and everyone else you know would be nice and content. And you'd all be lacking in energy and dying of boredom.

If you want to avoid stress totally you may as well start looking for a coffin. Feeling bored and unchallenged or stuck in a rut is just as draining mentally and emotionally as being burdened down with stress. You need a certain amount of

challenge and tension in your life to feel alive.
So if you're lacking in energy, take a careful look
at your life and see where you can give yourself
greater challenge and stimulation. Perhaps it's
time to learn a new language, review your career
or take up a new hobby? You should also pay
particular attention to the energy tips on
pages 171–74.

Pessimism

Negative mental and emotional states such as
fear, guilt, anger, anxiety, loneliness and worry
may be the biggest energy-drainers of them all,
increasing your risk not just of fatigue and
unhappiness but of poor health in general.
Although a positive attitude may not be a cure-
all, studies do suggest that patients who are
positive and optimistic experience fewer, less
severe symptoms and recover more quickly than
pessimistic, negative thinkers. People who think
positively also seem to have a better overall
quality of life.

Bear in mind that negativity in others can
also sap your strength. Listening to someone
you know complain or moan constantly about

the weather, their workload or life in general is a real downer. To preserve your energy, distance yourself from people like that as much as possible. If you can't, disarm them with your positive and upbeat approach. Although relationships with people who have a glass-half-empty approach to life can wear you out, don't forget that relationships with people who understand the importance of give and take can be a source of great happiness. The secret is to set boundaries and to learn to say 'no' when you are stretched too thinly.

Negative thoughts seem to breed and produce more negative thoughts, causing a downward spiral. If you tend to be a pessimist by nature, catch yourself whenever you have a negative thought and try to turn it around into a positive statement. It will be hard at first, but if you keep repeating the positive statements, they will begin to take hold and grow.

If you are prone to worry and negativity, as well as eating healthily and getting the mood-boosting effects of regular exercise (preferably in the fresh air), you should pay particular attention to the energy tips on pages 159-70.

Energy-draining medical conditions

For the great majority of people who suffer from low energy levels, diet and lifestyle factors are chiefly to blame. It is important to bear in mind, however, that many hidden diseases and disorders can also trigger fatigue.

Listed below are the conditions that are most commonly associated with low energy levels. If your fatigue interferes with the quality of your life for more than three weeks and can't be explained by diet and lifestyle habits, you should see a doctor without delay. This is particularly important if you are suffering from additional symptoms such as night sweats, weight change, breathlessness, pale mucous membranes in the nose and mouth, blood in faeces or urine, swollen lymph glands, irregular or absent periods, or constant thirst.

Fatigue is a good enough reason for you to seek your doctor's advice. Persistent fatigue should never be ignored in the hope that it will go away.

Iron-deficiency anaemia

Around 4 million women in the UK suffer from anaemia caused by lack of iron, but the syndrome may also occur in men.

Iron is essential to the formation of haemoglobin, the oxygen-carrying component of red blood cells. A nutritional deficiency of iron can lead to low blood haemoglobin levels and a reduced supply of oxygen to organs, tissues and cells. Inadequate oxygen supplies immediately inhibit your body's energy production and can result in fatigue, apathy, irritability, a racing heart rate and shortness of breath. In other words, your body needs iron to produce red blood cells and carry oxygen around your body; without it you'll feel lethargic no matter how much sleep you get.

If you suffer from tiredness and heavy periods, ask your doctor for a blood test to determine your iron levels. To reduce the risk of anaemia, make sure you eat a balanced diet with plenty of green vegetables. Don't take iron supplements unless advised to by your doctor, as the best way to get your iron is from your diet.

Undiagnosed diabetes

According to the Healthcare Commission, thousands of people in the UK may be unaware that they have diabetes. This is partly to do with high-sugar diets, obesity and sedentary lifestyles. Diabetes occurs when the amount of glucose (sugar) in your blood is too high and your body is unable to convert it into energy because there is not enough insulin or the insulin produced isn't working properly. The body then breaks down its stores of fat and protein to try to release more glucose, and the problem gets worse. This is why people with untreated diabetes can often feel tired and lose weight. Other symptoms include urinating often and extreme thirst.

To rule out diabetes, ask your doctor for a blood test. If the test is negative for diabetes then your tiredness might be caused by your blood sugar levels. Cravings for starchy, sweet or fatty foods can mean you have a blood sugar imbalance. To keep your blood sugar levels steady avoid sugar and refined, processed foods as well as juices, cigarettes and caffeine. Eat every 3 hours and load up on wholegrains, vegetables, legumes, nuts, seeds and foods that are as fresh, natural and as unprocessed as possible.

Underactive thyroid

Your thyroid works by producing the hormones which control metabolism and regulate energy levels. If your thyroid produces too little of these hormones, you feel tired. You might gain weight, your skin and hair will feel dry, and you may also feel depressed.

To rule out problems with your thyroid, ask your doctor for a thyroid test. If you have an underactive thyroid, he or she will prescribe medication to boost your hormone levels. You should also exercise regularly and eat a diet high in fruit, vegetables, fish and seaweed, while avoiding alcohol and cigarettes.

Food intolerances

One in 10 people in the UK has a food intolerance that can cause lethargy and irritability. Food intolerances trigger an immune response which uses up a huge amount of energy, and the most common food culprits are wheat, dairy products and sugar. So if your lunch was a cheese sandwich on wholewheat bread with a bar of chocolate, your body may be using up energy simply digesting your meal rather than converting it into energy.

If you suspect that you have a food intolerance, keep a food diary for a few weeks and see if there is a connection between your tiredness and a specific food. Common offenders are dairy products, soy, corn and gluten (found in wheat and other grains). Try eliminating the food that you suspect is making you feel tired and see if this makes a difference. Alternatively, you can ask your doctor to give you a blood test to check for food allergies.

Other common causes of fatigue
Sinusitis: An infection of the sinuses that is caused by irritation due to allergies, or by bacterial infection. Symptoms include stuffy nose, headache and fatigue, which are so similar to cold symptoms it can be hard to know what is going on. This perhaps explains why sinusitis is one of the most common causes of fatigue – millions of people suffer in silence.

PCOS (polycystic ovary syndrome):
If you're a woman and, despite eating healthily,
you find that the weight is piling on, you may be
suffering from PCOS, which can affect as many
as 1 in 5 women. Fatigue and weight gain are
symptoms of this under-diagnosed condition, in
which the ovaries and sometimes the adrenal
glands, for unknown reasons, pump out too much
male hormone. Thinning hair, insulin resistance,
excess facial hair, severe acne, irregular periods
and impaired fertility are other symptoms. To rule
out PCOS, make an appointment with your doctor
and discuss the possibility of PCOS as a cause for
your fatigue. If you are diagnosed with the
condition, the good news is that, as with diabetes
– and hypertension or high blood pressure –
PCOS can be successfully managed with a low
glycaemic diet and lifestyle changes. Patients
may also be considered for treatment with a
diabetes medicine called Metformin, especially if
they're overweight. It seems to reduce excess
male hormones and balance blood sugar levels.

Hypertension: Recent research has linked
sleep disorders and chronic tiredness to high
blood pressure. Like diabetes, high blood

pressure or hypertension is a silent disease, and you may not be aware that you have it. This is another reason why regular check-ups with your doctor or GP are advised.

Sleep apnoea: Sleep disorders such as sleep apnoea can seriously disrupt sleep and cause chronic fatigue during the day. A person with sleep apnoea has breathing problems when they are sleeping, and this can cause loud snoring and frequent night waking.

Chronic fatigue syndrome (CFS): CFS is a recognised medical condition that causes exhaustion and fatigue without any clear causal factors. There is no hard-and-fast test for this syndrome, but it is diagnosed 'by exclusion'. This means that if doctors have tested for everything else without success, this is the only possibility left. Chronic fatigue is nonetheless a real condition. Although it is not directly treatable, it can be managed well enough to allow people to return to good health in time.

Depression: One of the most common symptoms of depression is fatigue. If your energy is low from a busy lifestyle, you're generally going to recognise the value of what you are doing with your life, even if it is exhausting. The hallmarks of depression are feelings of helplessness, hopelessness and the inability to do anything about it. So if you start to feel that there is nothing you can do but give up and this feeling doesn't go away after two weeks, it's usually time to see your doctor or a therapist.

Medication: Many over-the-counter medications and prescription medicines have fatigue as a side effect. Antihistamines, beta-blockers, antidepressants and cholesterol medications, among others, could be causing tiredness, so if you are on any medication and are constantly feeling tired, be sure to make an appointment with your doctor to discuss the side effects of your medication and to suggest possible alternatives.

Weight gain: You probably don't need reminding that carrying excess weight increases your risk of heart disease, diabetes, aches and pains, and poor health in general. You may need reminding, however, that weight gain is a major cause of chronic tiredness. Carrying all that excess weight around is exhausting. If you need to lose weight, the first and most important rule is to never go on a diet. Crash diets, however tempting they may sound, are not the answer. Although you may lose weight initially, the chances are you'll end up putting it all back on again. Quick-fix and faddy diets don't teach you how to change your eating habits on a long-term basis, which is what you really need to do if you're going to keep the weight off. So forget about dieting, fad or otherwise, and think about a whole new way of eating.

Successful dieters are not people who are on a diet at all, but those who learn how to eat plenty of healthy, fresh food rich in nutrients that can boost their metabolism and energy, and who get plenty of energy-boosting exercise every day.

Clock change: Twice every year the clocks go either forward or back one hour. This can create problems falling asleep as it tinkers with your body clock. You may experience fatigue and loss of energy and symptoms similar to mild jet lag. To make the transition a little less tiring, begin to re-jig your sleeping routine a few days before the time change by hitting the sack earlier (for the Spring clock change) or later (for the Autumn change). You could start by going to bed 15 minutes earlier or later, and then the next night 30 minutes and so on. You could also reorganise your mealtime schedule by eating dinner earlier or later. Once the clocks have changed, get at least 15 minutes' exposure to sunlight, without glasses on, first thing in the morning. The bright sunlight (or any bright light) tells your body's natural biological clock that it's time to wake up; that same clock will then be set to tell your body it's time to go to sleep about 14 to 16 hours later. Finally, maintain an easier schedule on the Monday after the time change, and try to minimise driving on that day.

If in doubt about the cause of constant fatigue see your doctor. In the great majority of cases tiredness is not caused by an underlying illness, but if you don't know why you're always tired, it may be increasing your risk of becoming ill. More and more scientific studies are showing correlations between tiredness with a variety of serious diseases, including hypertension, diabetes, lupus and depression. So if your tiredness has gone on for more than two or three weeks, be sure to make an appointment with your doctor for a health check.

The energy solution

The causes of low energy can be many and varied, and getting a good night's sleep may not always provide the answer. In fact, getting too much sleep can be just as harmful as getting too little. However, if medical reasons for your tiredness have been ruled out and your energy is still persistently low, it is time to make simple but important changes to your diet and lifestyle.

Nothing has a more profound effect on your life than your energy. Remember, your energy levels are not determined at birth. They depend on what you eat and drink, and how you choose to think and live. You have more control of your zest levels than you think.

The 100 energy boosters that follow will help give you the right fuel and all the advice you need to reinvigorate yourself both in the short and long term. They will help you meet the demands and challenges of your daily life with energy and enthusiasm, and in the process improve your health, reduce stress, smooth out wrinkles and help you become a more energetic, relaxed and alive person.

PART TWO:

• •

100 ENERGY BOOSTERS

You don't have to work through the 100 energy boosters in any particular order; just dive into the sections that feel right to you. Whichever way you choose to incorporate them into your life, rest assured that each and every energy booster will bring out the latent but abundant energy resources within you.

Hopefully you will find enough suggestions and ideas in here to put the spring back into your step and the zest back into your life.

Boost energy with a good night's sleep

1 Beat the clock

Steady energy levels are among the acknowledged benefits of a good night's sleep. If you need an alarm clock to wake up in the morning, you aren't getting enough re-energising sleep. If, however, you can anticipate your alarm clock by waking up 5 to 30 minutes before it goes off feeling naturally refreshed, chances are you are getting a good night's sleep.

If you find it impossible to get out of bed without an alarm, don't change the time you rise. Instead, go to bed half an hour earlier than usual for the next week to give your biological clock a chance to reset. If you still need an alarm clock after a week, add 15 to 30 more minutes to your sleep time for another week. Keep going until you can wake without the alarm and feel alert and energetic all day.

2 Bounce out of bed
(at 7.22 a.m.)

Many of us try to make up for
lost sleep by staying in bed longer
on days off and weekends, but these lie-ins might
be doing you more harm than good. Your brain does
not have a different biological clock for weekdays
and weekends. If you have a long lie-in on Sunday
you are likely to stay up until the small hours of
Monday morning. A few hours later the alarm
clock will disturb your peaceful slumber and you'll
start your day feeling sleepy and fuzzy-headed.

Sleep experts believe that 6 to 8 hours' sleep is
optimum for most people. And if you want to enjoy
maximum health and vitality, your sleep must be
regular. This means getting up and going to bed
at the same time each day, including weekends.

So on days off, don't stay in bed. It's far
healthier to get up when you wake up naturally.
Research shows that those who get up early feel
more alert than those who rise later. In fact, 7.22
a.m. was the precise time experts pinpointed, so
– if you can – avoid burning the midnight oil and
let the morning sun shine in.

3 Make the most of doziness

In the few moments before you are fully awake, you're in what is called a 'hypnopompic state' – about the closest you can get to being hypnotised without nodding off. Your body is awake but your brain is highly suggestive to whatever thoughts you want to plant there. So turn on your back (you're less likely to fall asleep again in this position) and focus on three things you are looking forward to that day. Even if it is just your first cup of tea, focusing on small positives helps you start the day optimistic and full of energy.

It doesn't matter if you don't feel like bounding out of bed. Just think about what you have to look forward to that day or what you want to achieve, and then just get up. The thoughts you think on waking can set the tone for the whole day. Tell yourself it's going to be a wonderful day and good things are going to happen. It can seem an effort at first, but after a few attempts you will feel more in control of your life and more energised.

4 Bed MOT

A good night's sleep often depends on how comfortable your bed is. Studies show that, on average, people with uncomfortable beds sleep 1 to 2 hours less at night than those with comfortable beds.

If your bed is fewer than 8 years old, a mattress-topper – a comfortable, supportive layer that sits on top of your mattress – can be the perfect solution. If your bed is older than 8, it will definitely need replacing.

When buying a new mattress, check that it supports your body at all points. If you aren't getting enough support you'll get back pain, but a mattress that's too hard can create uncomfortable pressure. There is nothing wrong with a soft mattress as long as it gives you enough support, especially in the small of your back and under your knees. The ideal mattress should keep your spine in alignment and distribute pressure evenly across your body. A mattress has to be soft enough to fill in the gap under your lower back, but not so soft that it sags completely under your weight.

5 Pillow talk

For good sleep comfort, you need the right pillow. Pillows should provide support for your neck and spine, alleviating pain that contributes to a poor night's sleep.

In general, the 'comfort lifetime' of a pillow ranges between 6 months (polyester pillows) and 5 years (down and feather pillows). If yours is showing clear signs of wear and tear, it needs replacing. If you aren't sure, test the support of down and feather pillows by laying the fluffed pillow on a hard surface. Fold it in half or thirds and squeeze out the air. Release the pillow. If it unfolds and returns to its original position, it still has support; a broken pillow will stay folded. To test the support of polyester pillows, fluff and fold as above. Then place a weight of around 280 g (10 oz) (a trainer is fine) on the pillow. A pillow with support will unfold itself and throw off the shoe; a worn-out pillow will stay folded.

When buying a new pillow, the best for you will be the one you can squish and fluff to meet your contours and sleeping position. You also need a pillow firm enough so there is no gap between it and your neck.

6 Roll over

If you're used to a certain sleeping position but that position isn't maximising your chances of waking refreshed in the morning, then it's time to get out of your comfort zone and try something different. Experts tend to recommend sleeping on your side with your spine straight, or on your back maintaining the natural curve of the spine, as these positions minimise the risk of sleep-disrupting aches and pains.

If you sleep on your side to maintain the natural curve of your spine, place a pillow between your bent knees to support your hips, and make sure your head pillow supports both your head and neck while keeping them in alignment.

If you sleep on your back, place a pillow under your knees to maintain the natural curve of your spine. If you sleep on your stomach, this position has the greatest potential to cause problems because it exaggerates the arch at the base of your spine, thereby causing strain. If you must sleep in this position, be sure to slightly raise one side of your body and place a pillow under your stomach.

7 Take a power nap

Studies have shown that a well-timed nap can greatly improve your ability to pay close attention to detail and make critical decisions. In today's hectic world, enjoying some shut-eye come mid-afternoon could well be one of the most powerful energy boosters of them all.

Many people experience a natural drowsiness in the afternoon, about eight hours after waking. It seems that this post-lunch dip is a normal part of the body's circadian rhythm and coincides with a slight drop in our body temperature. Research in countries such as Spain and Italy, where people have a sleep mid-afternoon, shows that you can make yourself more alert, reduce stress and improve brain function with a well-timed nap.

Naps aren't necessary if you are getting enough sleep at night and don't feel tired during the day. If you do feel tired in the afternoon, though, and have a dip in energy, you would benefit from a nap. Here are some guidelines:

Prime nap time is 1 – 3 p.m.

Optimum nap time is 20 minutes. Any more than that and your nap will take you into a deeper stage of sleep, and you will most likely wake up feeling groggy rather than energised.

Find a quiet place where you won't be disturbed and set your alarm to go off 20 minutes later. Make yourself as comfortable as you can. Lying down would be great, but if this isn't possible rest your head on a table or lie back in a chair with your shoes off. Your body temperature falls when you sleep, so cover yourself with a blanket.

Try to create a consistent routine. You shouldn't nap just once or twice a week; you have to do it on a daily basis or you'll upset your circadian rhythm and have problems sleeping at night.

If you really haven't got time for a nap, try switching off for a few moments instead. Daydreaming gives your body a rest and produces the slower brainwaves that occur during regular sleep.

8 Pull those socks up

During the night your temperature drops before you fall asleep, rises during the night and then falls again before you wake. So if you wear heavy or tight-fitting clothes to bed, you could wake up in the middle of the night in a hot sweat. It seems the only exception to this rule is wearing socks. Because your feet have the poorest circulation, they often feel colder than the rest of your body, and research has shown that people who wear bed socks fall asleep more quickly and have a better night's sleep than those with bare feet.

Wear whatever is comfortable for you to bed, or sleep in the buff. Bear in mind that cotton T-shirts or pyjamas are most likely to stop you waking up feeling hot and uncomfortable. So always think lighter rather than heavier when buying bedclothes. The key should be comfort over style, so choose something that is loose-fitting and moves with you properly during sleep, even if it is a size bigger than you normally wear. Keeping your neck and shoulders warm is important, so you may want to change into something else if you wear a negligee.

9 Use the power of the dark side

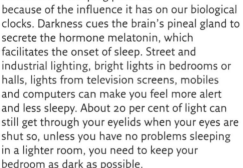

Scientists have discovered that natural daylight has the greatest effect on our sleeping patterns because of the influence it has on our biological clocks. Darkness cues the brain's pineal gland to secrete the hormone melatonin, which facilitates the onset of sleep. Street and industrial lighting, bright lights in bedrooms or halls, lights from television screens, mobiles and computers can make you feel more alert and less sleepy. About 20 per cent of light can still get through your eyelids when your eyes are shut so, unless you have no problems sleeping in a lighter room, you need to keep your bedroom as dark as possible.

Dim the lights as you prepare to go to sleep to help you unwind. Turn your clock radio away so that it does not shine directly at you. Light-blocking shades, lined drapes and even an eye mask can ensure that light doesn't interfere with your sleep, thereby increasing your chances of waking up refreshed and energised.

10 Silent night

Sounds of more than 45 decibels – the volume of someone talking quietly – can wake you up, but even sounds as low as 20 decibels can interfere with the quality of your sleep. If you find your sleep disrupted by noises such as the screech of sirens, the rumble of trains, the rise and fall of conversation, airplanes overhead, a dog's barking or a partner's snoring, then consider buying earplugs.

Ear canals are very much like fingerprints – no two are alike. So the best thing if you want to use earplugs is to experiment with several different brands to establish which are most comfortable. Foam earplugs are inserted by first rolling the plug between thumb and index finger to squash the foam into a thin tube, then placing it in your ear and holding it there until the foam has fully expanded. Some people prefer wax earplugs, believing that they give a 'snugger' fit. Whichever you choose, a properly sized and inserted plug will be comfortable for a full night's sleep and should be able to block out distracting noises.

11 Sleep apart, together

If your partner snores, talks or kicks in his or her sleep, or has different sleep needs and routines to you, consider sleeping in a separate bedroom.

Research by the UK Sleep Council found that one in four of us frequently retreats to a spare room or sofa for a restful and refreshing night's sleep. This often has nothing to do with a problem in the relationship and everything to do with an urgent need for a good night's sleep.

If you decide to sleep apart, this isn't a sign that your relationship is in trouble; quite the opposite. Studies show that people who sleep poorly have a higher divorce rate. With a good night's sleep you have more energy to devote to your relationship.

If sleeping in separate rooms isn't possible for whatever reason, try the following:

If your partner snores, encourage them to use a nasal spray or strip. You could also wear earplugs or go to bed before them so that you are already asleep when they come to bed.

If your partner kicks and shoves, buy a bigger bed or put two single mattresses together. If you never win the duvet war, invest in separate duvets.

12 Sweet dreams

When you were a child the chances
are your parents established a bedtime
routine for you. They may have given
you a warm bath, read you a story and then
settled you in bed. All of these things helped you
drift off to sleep. A routine helped then, and it
can help now.

Establishing a familiar routine and treating
the last half an hour before bedtime with calm
and respect will also help you learn to place a
value on sleep. If you want to enjoy life to the
full and have the energy you need to be wide
awake, alert and at your best all day long, you
need to respect the need of your body and your
mind for rest.

A bedtime routine can be the key to a good
night's sleep, but the secret is to find what
works best for you. Whatever you decide, keep
things as gentle, friendly and calm as possible in
your bedroom, especially in the last half hour
before you go to bed.

Reading, chatting to friends, writing in a
journal and other calming activities are all

recommended just before sleep. Many people find that a cup of herbal tea or warm milk has a relaxing effect.

Some gentle stretching or yoga exercises before bedtime can relax body and mind, but don't do anything vigorous and avoid exercising for three hours before bedtime. Exercising later than this (unless it's sex) may disturb your sleep.

Just before going to bed, soak yourself in a warm, relaxing bath. This will send the blood away from your brain to your skin surface and make you feel both relaxed and drowsy.

If you fall asleep the moment your head hits the pillow, you need to go to bed earlier as it should take you around 10–15 minutes to drift off. There will, however, be nights when you simply can't get to sleep. When this happens don't lie there getting anxious or frustrated; get out of bed until you feel drowsy again. Try to stay in surroundings that are dimly lit and do some light reading or some repetitive task that does not require a lot of brain work, like light housework. The chances are it won't take long before you feel sleepy and want to return to your warm bed.

13 Great bedroom design

It's really important to associate your bedroom with pleasure and rest. Creating the right atmosphere in the bedroom can help you sleep more soundly, and – as we have seen – sound sleep is the foundation of well-balanced energy levels.

Create a sleep-conductive environment that is dark, quiet, comfortable, cool and free of interruptions; these are the conditions you need for sleep. Select colours that you associate with peace and calm. Many people choose green or blue because it reminds them of the sea or of nature. Or go for pastel shades that are easy and gentle on the eye.

In general, make your bedroom reflect the value you place on sleep and use it only for sleep and sexual activity, not for watching TV, eating, working or surfing the 'net. Clear out clutter, TVs and other electrical appliances, and hide illuminated clocks from view or cover them with a cloth to avoid clockwatching at night. Finally, a slightly cool room is optimum for good sleep, so aim for around 16–18°C (62–65°F).

Boost energy with food

14 Freedom from transfats

Banned in Denmark, compulsorily labelled in the US and linked to cardiovascular disease and weight gain – transfatty acid must go. If you ditch the transfats you will eat less of the junk that clogs your system and leaves you feeling sluggish, tired and bloated. In the long term you can also stave off high cholesterol.

Most manufactured foods have transfats in them, including margarine, cakes, pies, biscuits, some vegetable oils and ready meals, as well as cheap chocolate, confectionary and ice cream. Instead of margarine it might be better to go for a small amount of butter instead. Watch out too for 'hydrogenated fats' – this is the nutritional term for transfats. If you've been upping your intake of whole foods and fibre, and cutting down on sugar and refined carbohydrates, you may have already cut down on the transfats in your diet.

15 Discover the zest

There's a reason nutritionists tend to recommend lemon juice as the first drink of the morning. If you've ever been to a health farm, or to India for that matter, you'll know that lemon juice is typically drunk immediately on waking. The reason is that lemon juice is a wonderful digestive aid. If your digestive system isn't functioning optimally it doesn't matter how many so-called 'super foods' you eat, you won't be getting the 'good-for-you' nutrients your body needs to produce energy.

Lemon juice, being a digestion-boosting power-house with an energising tangy flavour, is therefore exactly the right drink to kickstart both your metabolism and your energy levels first thing. So, as soon as you wake up – before getting dressed or having breakfast – drink a glass of lemon juice.

Energy-boosting lemonade

2 tbsp freshly squeezed lemon juice
  (approx. ½ to 1 lemon)
300–500 ml (10–17 fl oz) pure filtered
  water
2 tsp organic maple syrup
Pinch of cayenne pepper, to taste

Mix all the ingredients together and drink
immediately.

Use fresh lemons only, and mix your
lemonade just before drinking. Adding a
pinch of cayenne pepper adds extra zing
to the flavour as well as a stimulatory
heating effect that speeds cleansing and
elimination. Maple syrup adds a sweet
taste for those who find the drink too bitter,
and boasts a welcome shot of zinc and
magnesium to help regulate your appetite
and further boost energy production.

16 Dynamic breakfasts

A mobile phone needs
recharging regularly so that
its battery doesn't run down,
and it's the same with your body. When you wake
up in the morning your body has been without
food for many hours and it needs refuelling.

The old cliché about breakfast being the most
important meal is true. Brains need a regular
supply of glucose to function, and in the
morning there isn't much glucose up there, so
never skip breakfast. If you do you are likely to
hit an energy wall at around 10 a.m. Eating
breakfast will boost your energy first thing and
help stop your stores of energy – your blood
sugar – from dipping during the morning. In
other words, it will give your body and mind the
energy they need to function optimally, setting
you up for the day ahead.

Eating breakfast also kickstarts your metabolism (fat-burning), so if you have weight to lose,
skipping breakfast is one of the biggest mistakes
you can make. You need to get your metabolism
up and running as soon as possible so that it

isn't on hold during the day and clinging onto the fat reserves you don't need.

You may not feel like eating 2 minutes after you jump out of bed, so give yourself a little time to wake up before eating. And don't just grab any food for breakfast; you need to make sure that what you are eating is optimum fuel for your body and brain. Avoid energy-draining fry-ups, coffee, white bread and muffins and sugary cereals with colourings made from refined grains. Make energy-boosting choices instead.

Dynamic breakfast choices include:

- A bowl of high-fibre cereal that is low in fat, sugar and salt with milk and a glass of fresh fruit juice.
- A boiled egg and wholemeal toast with a glass of fresh fruit juice.
- Oat porridge topped with bananas and fresh and dried fruit, and green or herbal tea

For rushed mornings, a fruit or protein. smoothie can be made the night before. In the morning just shake it up and drink as you get ready to start your day.

17 Avoid the rush

The typical way many of us find ourselves eating is a small or non-existent breakfast followed by a light snack during the day and a big meal at night. Sometimes people don't eat anything at all until their evening meal which can be as late as 8.30 p.m. Stacking your calories like this isn't a good idea and will almost certainly lead to fatigue and energy-draining weight gain.

In the fasted state your body will reduce your metabolism (fat-burning) and then – when you do eat before you go to bed – your body has little opportunity to produce energy and burn any of the calories that have been consumed. The result: poor digestion, weight gain and fatigue.

For sustained energy release you should start the day with a healthy breakfast, have a mid-morning snack, then lunch, a mid-afternoon snack and then supper. Eating every few hours will avoid a rush of blood sugar followed by a low, keeping your blood sugar levels and your energy levels as stable as possible. It doesn't have to be anything more than a piece of fruit and a handful of nuts and seeds. The important thing is to avoid going for long hours on nothing more than a cup of coffee and a chocolate bar.

For steady energy release, try to make the basis of your daily meal pattern a healthy proportion of unrefined carbohydrates (fruits, vegetables, grains, legumes) and a little protein (dairy produce, nuts and seeds) to keep your blood sugars balanced, together with a modest amount of dietary fat. It is an excellent idea to avoid sources of saturated fat from red meat, fried and fatty fast foods, cakes, pastries and crisps, and to concentrate on obtaining omega-3 and omega-6 essential fats from oily fish, nuts, seeds, extra-virgin olive oil and sunflower oil. Contrary to popular belief a healthy diet is not fat free. For steady energy release you need a constant and daily supply of essential fats to keep your calorie burn high, your skin smooth, your brain alert and your body healthy.

18 Raw potential

Eat something raw at the start of every meal.
By eating foods in their natural state you can
access their valuable energy-boosting nutrients
more easily. So, without going overboard, begin
each meal with something raw – for example an
apple at breakfast, a stick of celery or some
chopped cucumber with lemon juice and olive
oil at lunch or supper.

Cooking generally causes nutrient loss, which
leads to fatigue. The more a food is cooked –
especially vegetables – the higher its sugar
content. Proteins, too, aren't spared by cooking.
When protein is overcooked it is destroyed.

This doesn't mean you shouldn't cook at all.
Certain foods such as eggs, meat and fish can be
dangerous to eat raw and need to be cooked
thoroughly. Try to balance cooked food with
more raw food: perhaps 50:50, and cook gently,
at a lower heat and for longer if necessary.
Steaming is the best way to cook veggies, stir-
frying is good for fish, and poaching is useful for
eggs and fish. Meat should be roasted since
other methods, such as frying, use too much fat.

19 The big chew

Most people think that digestion begins in the stomach, but it actually begins in the mouth. The process of chewing is a vital component of good digestion, and therefore of good health and steady energy levels.

Avoid eating on the run. You need to chew your food thoroughly if you are to digest it properly and get the maximum benefit from what you eat. So don't eat at your desk while working, and try to avoid grabbing a bite to eat as you run from one appointment to another. Make time to ensure that you eat a proper meal rather than just the fuel you need as quickly as possible.

The next time you have a meal or snack, concentrate on noticing every morsel: what it looks, smells and tastes like. Count to five between each bite, or put your knife and fork down between bites. It doesn't really take much time or effort to chew your food, and what you get in return is better digestion, better health, more energy and a greater enjoyment and appreciation of food.

20 Power in a pot

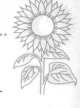

In recent years the term 'probiotics' has become a health buzzword, as several research studies have pointed to its health- and digestion-boosting benefits.

There are trillions of bacteria in your digestive tract and not all of them are good for you. However, about 10 per cent of your body's energy is created by the healthy bacteria in your gut. If you have enough of the healthy bacteria, they can be your first line of defence against unhealthy bacteria and other viruses that inhibit digestion, lower immunity and drain your energy. The healthy, energy-boosting bacteria are known as probiotics; the three main ones are *Lactobacillus acidophilus*, *Lactobacillus salivarius* and those in the genus *Bifidobacterium*. All of these have been shown to reduce the levels of unhealthy bacteria, repair intestinal lining and inhibit disease-promoting microbes.

Energy-boosting probiotic supplements are available from health food stores. However, unless you've been suffering from an infection and need to give your digestive tract a boost, or have been diagnosed a course of probiotics by a nutritionist, there's really no need to take a probiotic supplement every day. It's much better for you to get your probiotic fix from fermented food sources such as miso, sourdough bread and sauerkraut, and pots of 'live' natural yoghurt containing *Lactobacillus acidophilus*.

With stress, pollution and antibiotic use wiping out friendly bacteria and draining our energy, we could all benefit from probiotics. Friendly bacteria survive about a week in the gut, so try to eat bio-yoghurt frequently, at least every other day. To prevent the bacteria being killed by stomach acid it is best eaten on its own rather than as a dessert. Alternatively, try one 15 minutes before a meal. If you are a vegan or dairy intolerant you can take probiotic supplements. Another way to boost good bacteria in our bodies is to eat foods known as 'prebiotics' that feed them. Bananas, barley, fruit, onions and soya beans are all prebiotics that can nourish and support good bacteria and by doing so, boost your health and your energy.

21 Energy elixirs

When you have a mid-morning or a mid-afternoon energy slump, don't reach for a sugar fix, coffee or a carbonated drink. All of these will unsettle your blood sugar levels and give you an initial high followed by that nasty slump. Energy bars aren't much better either, as they don't provide much more energy than other food with the same amount of calories, and are likely to be lower in nutrients. Make use of freshly prepared fruit smoothies instead.

Although fruit does contain natural sweetness in the form of fructose, it is less likely to give you a violent sugar rush because the fibre in fruit stops it entering your blood stream too rapidly. Fruit also contains crucial nutrients such as antioxidant vitamins that can give your immune system a boost. The following are some suggestions for simple combinations of fruit smoothies. Use them as a basis for experiment and to discover energy elixirs of your own:

Banana brilliance: Put 250 ml (8 fl oz) natural live yoghurt, 1 large or 2 small ripe bananas, 1 tsp grade B maple syrup and a few drops of vanilla essence extract to taste in a blender. Blend until smooth.

Orange pick-me-up: A smoothie made with tea gives an energy boost but at far less strength than a cup of coffee. In addition it won't dehydrate you as much or deplete your body of energy-boosting nutrients. Put 1 large orange, peeled and cut into pieces, 125 ml (4 fl oz) iced tea, 200 ml (7 fl oz) orange sorbet and 3 ice cubes in a blender and blend until smooth.

Berry energiser: 250 ml (8 fl oz) milk, 3 or 4 sweet strawberries, half a ripe banana and a dash of clear organic honey. Blend until smooth.

Amazing apricot: 5 fresh apricots, 375 ml natural live yoghurt, a taste of clear honey and a splash of milk (to lighten the texture, if necessary). Blend until smooth.

Honey and banana surprise: 2 large peeled oranges, 1 ripe peeled banana, 1 tsp grade B maple syrup and a handful of ice. Blend and enjoy.

22 Go to work on an egg

Eggs are a nutrient-packed high-protein food that have been wrongly maligned for their cholesterol content. We need some cholesterol to make sex hormones, along with the stress hormones necessary for handling our busy lives. Eggs are also good brain food as they are packed with choline, needed for healthy brain cells and to make the memory messenger acetylcholine. You can eat up to seven eggs a week, boiled or poached, but not fried. An egg is only as healthy as the chicken it came from, so try to buy organic.

Sardines also contain choline, so eat them at least once a week, grilled with lemon juice or even out of a tin on wholemeal toast.

23 Raise your glass

Your body is made up of two-thirds water, so water intake and distribution are crucial for good health and energy. Water helps keep your blood sugar and hormones balanced, as well as helping your body to eliminate waste. It also keeps your skin glowing and your cells working properly, while delivering energy-boosting nutrients to all of your organs.

If you don't drink enough water you will start to feel dizzy and tired, so to keep your energy levels high drink pure (filtered if necessary) water throughout the day, even if you don't feel thirsty. If you are feeling thirsty, you are already dehydrated. In all, you should be aiming to drink 6 to 8 glasses a day, more if you are exercising, if you are under extra physical or emotional stress, or if it is very hot and you are losing fluids through perspiration.

Tea, coffee, caffeinated drinks and alcohol do not count as they sap your energy and deplete your body of nutrients. Water is the best drink for quenching thirst and hydrating the body to prevent fatigue, dry skin, headaches and sore eyes.

24 Sweet alternatives

If you're craving something sweet to give you a quick energy boost, you can avoid the sugar blues by trying the following sweet alternatives.

Go for fresh or dried fruits such as apricots, apples or pears. Fruit is power-packed with nutrients that can give you a natural and sustained energy boost.

A pot of live natural yoghurt with fruit is a sweet, creamy, satisfying and nutritious alternative.

Instead of guzzling a fizzy drink loaded with sugar, try a fruit smoothie instead, made from the juices of real fruits.

Try a bowl of hot oat cereal with a pinch of cinnamon or maple syrup on top. It will satisfy your sweet tooth, keep hunger at bay, boost your metabolism and give you a comfort fix at the same time.

A small bar of quality dark chocolate (at least 70 per cent cocoa) is naturally rich in energy-boosting antioxidants. In moderation it can offer chocoholics a healthy alternative to high-sugar chocolate bars.

25 Green is the new black

Cut down on caffeine until you're only having around 300 ml (½ pint) a day. Although coffee pumps you up, it also lets you down and, if drunk in the afternoon, can keep you awake at night.

One of the best alternatives to black tea or coffee is green tea. Studies have shown that green tea has only a quarter of the amount of caffeine as coffee, and it can actually help boost energy and weight loss. The reason is that green tea contains substances called catechins which can boost metabolism (fat-burning) and activate brain chemicals. Some people may feel a lift after just one cup of green tea, while others need more; four cups is a good daily limit.

Apart from green tea and red tea, which is also lower in caffeine than coffee, there are a number of good coffee substitutes. These are grain-based formulas made from roasted barley with added flavourings.

You can also choose from a huge range of refreshing herbal or fruit teas. Good energy-boosting herbal tea choices include ginger, lemon grass, peppermint, apple and orange blossom.

26 Eat a rainbow

Raw, fresh vegetables and fruits play a major role in boosting health and energy. Dark green, orange, red and yellow fruits and vegetables, in particular, are packed with antioxidants that can help boost immunity and slow down ageing. If you want to maximize the benefits that come from antioxidants, make a point of including a wide variety of fruits and vegetables in your diet every day. One way to do this is to make sure that there is plenty of natural colour on your plate.

The more natural colour on your plate, the more likely the food you are eating contains high concentrations of energy-boosting vitamins, minerals and other micronutrients your body needs.

Naturally coloured fruits and vegetables not only supply sustained energy but they can also reduce your chances of developing some types of cancer, diabetes or heart disease. Five to eight servings a day, depending on your energy needs, are part of the foundation of a healthy diet. Mix and match some of each of the following colours daily for the best results:

Yellow and orange: provide vitamin C, folate, betacarotene and carotenoids that can boost immunity, help your eyesight and make your skin glow. Think mangoes and sweet potatoes.

Purple and blue: contain anthocyanins to help protect against cancer and heart disease. Think blueberries and blackberries.

White: contain allicin, which can help lower blood pressure and cholesterol. Think cauliflower, garlic and onions.

Red: contain lycopene, an antioxidant that can help fight cancer. Think tomatoes and watermelon.

Green: contain fibre, minerals and antioxidants to boost your immunity. Think spinach, rocket, asparagus, watercress and broccoli. Green vegetables are also packed with detoxifying nutrients. A happy liver means more energy, clearer skin and brighter eyes, so try to aim for two servings of green vegetables daily, in addition to your usual five portions. Adding some vinegar or lemon juice to your vegetables and salad will also give your liver an added boost, as vinegar helps its functioning by manufacturing more bile.

27 Full of beans

Beans are the best possible food for satisfying hunger and giving you stamina.

Warm bean salad
250 g (8 oz) okra, finely sliced
2 large garlic cloves, crushed
175 ml (6 fl oz) water
175 g 6 oz) tinned butter beans, drained
175 g (6 oz) tinned red kidney beans, drained
2 tsp lemon juice; 2 tsp extra-virgin olive oil
Large handful of mixed herbs
Handful of walnuts
2 thick slices crusty wholemeal bread

1 Put the okra, garlic and water into a saucepan, cover and bring to the boil. Reduce heat and simmer gently for 3 minutes until soft. Drain.
2 In a separate saucepan, gently heat the beans with the lemon juice for 20 minutes.
3 Strain, then add okra, garlic, oil, herbs and walnuts to taste. Stir gently and serve with the bread.

28 Do the protein shake

Protein gives your body an even supply of energy, as well as the amino acids it needs to build and repair muscles, and manufacture hormones and brain cells. It also has a stabilising effect on blood sugar, producing steady long-term energy.

Good sources of protein include oily fish, nuts, seeds, legumes, dairy products and grains. Ideally your protein intake should be split throughout the day. Vegetarians and vegans need to be especially careful that they get enough protein in their diet; they should substitute pulses, legumes, wholegrains, dairy products, tofu, eggs, nuts, seeds or Quorn instead.

DIY protein shake
Handful of fresh blueberries
Handful of fresh raspberries
150 g (5 oz) live yoghurt
150 ml (¼ pint) soya milk; 50 g (2 oz) muesli
Small handful ice cubes

Place all the ingredients in a blender and enjoy!

29 Pass on the sugar

Foods that are high in refined sugar may taste good and give you an instant energy boost, but it comes at a very high price. Sugar that isn't used up immediately by your body for energy gets converted to fat, something most of us want to avoid. The solution is simple: to avoid the sugar rush, boost your energy and trim your waistline, you've got to pass on the sugar.

> **Sugar shutdown action plan**
> ✔ **Cut down on foods with added sugar:** Sweets, biscuits, pies and other processed foods contain added sugar.
> ✔ **Cut down on refined foods:** Foods such as white bread, white rice, instant potato and cornflakes act like sugar in your system because they lack fibre. It's always best to stick with wholegrains and fresh fruits and vegetables for a steady release of sugar. Forget the glycaemic index: the fastest way to work out the impact a food is going to have on your blood sugar is to

think about how refined it is. If it is highly refined and contains lots of sugar, salt, additives and preservatives, it's going to upset your blood sugar levels and trigger fatigue.

✔ **Ditch low fat:** Many foods advertised as low fat make up for it by being very high in sugar. It's actually better to eat the full-fat versions in moderation than to overload on low-fat, high-sugar ones.

✔ **Check the label:** Start checking food labels, as sugar is a hidden ingredient in many foods and has different names including concentrated fruit juice, corn syrup, glucose, lactose, maltose and sucrose. Avoid artificial sweeteners, too, as they have been linked to weight gain and headaches. If you really need sweetness, it's much better to add fruit or spices such as cinnamon and nutmeg.

✔ **Keep on snacking:** You might find it hard if you have a sweet tooth to cut down at first, but if you are eating every few hours you'll find that sweet cravings naturally recede because your blood sugars are stable.

30 Energy day

Maximise your energy by following this 24-hour energy-boosting meal plan the day before an important event, such as a presentation or exam.

On rising: Glass of lemon juice.

Breakfast: Piece of fruit; two scrambled eggs with one slice of rye bread or sugar-free muesli with fresh fruit, live yoghurt and soya milk. Glass of fruit juice.

Snack mid-morning: Two pieces of fresh fruit; a palmful of mixed seeds. Cup of green tea.

Lunch: High-energy spinach soup (*see* page 87); grilled, steamed or stir-fried chicken, tofu or fish with three portions of vegetables; one serving of brown rice.

Snack mid-afternoon: Raw vegetables or fruit, with glass of soya milk. Cup of ginger tea.

Dinner: Choose a different protein from the one you had at lunch; two portions of fresh vegetables with warm bean salad.

Make sure you drink at least 6 to 8 glasses of water during the day and avoid all high-sugar foods and drinks.

31 Be an iron lady or lord

Iron helps your blood cells carry oxygen needed for energy. Getting the right amount of iron can improve your performance and productivity at work and at home.

The following are all good sources of iron:

✔ whole grain cereals and bread
✔ green vegetables
✔ dried fruit such as apricots or raisins
✔ nuts and seeds such as cashews or almonds
✔ lentils, peas and beans.

Iron supplements aren't necessary unless your doctor advises them, but try to include iron-rich foods in your diet every day to reduce your risk of anaemia (a condition that occurs when you don't have enough healthy red blood cells).

Foods high in vitamin C help your body absorb iron more efficiently, so eat foods such as citrus fruits and juices, cantaloupe melons, strawberries, tomatoes and dark green vegetables along with iron-rich foods to boost both flavour and nutrition. Choose breads, cereals and pastas that say 'enriched' or 'iron-fortified' on the label. If your cereal isn't fortified, adding a handful or raisins will up the iron content.

32 Mighty magnesium

When you are magnesium deficient your bodily functions slow down at the cellular level, causing everything to become sluggish until eventually fatigue ensues. It has been suggested that Chronic Fatigue Syndrome is related to persistent magnesium deficiency and may improve with a magnesium-enriched diet.

People who suffer from an unusual amount of anxiety have been found to have lower levels of magnesium. Other studies have found that magnesium supplements reduce the release and effect of stress hormones on the heart. Evidence also suggests that magnesium may play an important role in regulating blood pressure, due to its natural muscle-relaxant ability.

Excellent sources of magnesium include spinach, grapes, mustard greens, summer squash, broccoli, blackstrap molasses, halibut, turnip greens, pumpkin seeds, cucumber, green beans, celery, kale and a variety of seeds including sunflower seeds, sesame seeds and flaxseeds.

33 Get hooked on fish (or flaxseeds)

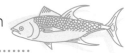

Without sufficient quantities of omega-3 and omega-6 EFAs (essential fats), your energy levels are going to dip. This is because these essential fats have a protective effect on your heart and give you improved brain function, as well as healthy hair and joints and smooth skin. They are, in addition, one of the best blood sugar stabilisers around, and stable blood sugar levels mean less likelihood of fatigue, mood swings, heart disease and weight gain.

All oily fish are a source of these important fats. They keep blood flowing smoothly, which delivers oxygen, energising cells and boosting your libido. Aim to eat oily fish at least twice a week – but not more than four times a week. If you don't eat fish you can eat sea vegetables (seaweed) and up your intake of hemp and flaxseeds – great sources of omega-3. You might like to try a daily dose of 3 tsp cold-pressed flaxseed oil or 3 tbsp ground flaxseeds. You can also use hemp and flaxseeds in salad dressings and smoothies.

✔ **Tip: Try sweet potato mashed with ginger for added zing.**

Sweet potatoes or yams are packed with energy-boosting minerals – calcium for strong bones, magnesium and potassium for energy production, as well as folic acid and the antioxidant immune-boosting vitamin C. Their complex carbohydrate and fibre content also has a steadying effect on blood sugar, ensuring that your energy supply is constant throughout the day.

✔ **Tip: Make a fruit salad every day with a variety of different coloured fruits, adding some freshly squeezed orange juice and a little cinnamon or ginger for a twist.**

Fruit is a great energy booster because it's a natural source of carbohydrates. Fruit is low in fat (the exception being avocado) and rich in a myriad of antioxidants and other health-enhancing nutrients such as fibre. Fruit is a great snack to be enjoyed at any time of day.

✔ Tip: Use different herbs and spices to add flavour to rice.

Rice is another great source of energy-giving carbohydrates. It is also extremely low in fat and contains many vitamins and minerals, including the B group vitamins thiamine and niacin, iron, zinc and magnesium. Brown rice is a richer source of these nutrients and is also a good source of dietary fibre.

✔ Tip: Try to use healthy sauces with your pasta, such as spinach and ricotta, and keep portion sizes small if you don't want to gain weight.

Pasta is another low-fat, carbohydrate-rich energy food that has become a staple in many people's diets. There are over 600 different types of pasta, including: spaghetti, fettuccine, ravioli, tortellini, linguini, gnocchi, macaroni and many more. These are characterised by their different forms and shapes, but nutritionally they are all very similar, providing plenty of carbohydrate, some protein, dietary fibre and vitamins, and minerals including the B group vitamins thiamine and niacin, iron and magnesium.

35 Eat your spinach

Popeye got it right – studies have
shown that eating two servings a
day of foods like tomatoes, leafy green
vegetables such as spinach and romaine lettuce,
pinto, navy or kidney beans and grain products
decreases levels of amino acid that contribute to
cardiovascular problems.

Although spinach can help build stamina and
boost energy because of its high nutrient
content, many people don't eat enough of it.
But researchers from the University of Arkansas
have come up with an easy solution – instead of
iceberg lettuce, put spinach in your sandwiches.
You won't taste the difference.

High-energy spinach soup (Serves 2)

1 tbsp olive oil
1 shallot, thinly sliced
1 leek, thinly sliced
1 small potato, diced
600 ml (1 pint) water
1 sprig fresh thyme or a heaped tsp of
    dried thyme
300 g (10 oz) fresh baby leaf spinach

1 Heat the oil in a heavy-bottomed pan on a medium heat. Add the shallot, leek and potato and soften for 5 minutes. Add the water, bring to the boil and simmer gently for about 30 minutes, ensuring the soup doesn't come to the boil.
2 Add the thyme and then the spinach, raising the heat slightly. Stir continuously for 4 minutes until the spinach leaves are dark green and limp. Take off the heat and leave the soup to stand for 15 minutes.
3 Blend the soup in a food processor until completely smooth. Reheat until hot but not boiling. Serve immediately with warm croutons and grated cheese.

36 Power lunch or dinner

....

We often hear that a good
breakfast contributes to how well
we feel and perform in the morning, but we also
need to refuel at lunchtime to make it through
the afternoon in top form! Consider energy
sandwiches, made by spreading two pieces of
wholemeal bread with any of the following:

✔ avocado, sliced chicken breast, sliced tomato,
   baby spinach, grated cheese
✔ cottage cheese and cucumber slices
✔ hummus, sliced tomato and watercress
✔ smoked tofu, cucumber and cress
✔ hard-boiled egg with cress, tomato and
   lettuce.

Eat with a portion of fresh vegetable soup.

A baked potato is another great foundation
for a power lunch, and sweet potatoes make a
delicious change. Have them with any of the
fillings below and a large salad:

✔ hummus with cucumber
✔ baked beans
✔ tuna in brine with 1 tsp cottage cheese.

37 Optimise feel-good brain chemicals

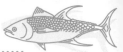

Gaining energy is not simply about physically fuelling your body. It also involves optimising levels of feel-good brain chemicals such as dopamine, which help to keep you fresh, upbeat and positive. Dopamine, made from the protein building-block tyrosine, is important for a healthy sex drive in women and men. When your dopamine levels dip, you are more likely to feel depressed, irritable and moody, and to experience loss of libido. Along with tyrosine, nutrients such as the B vitamin folic acid, vitamin B12 and magnesium provide the foundation for dopamine production.

Steak, lean lamb, pork, chicken, pheasant, turkey, venison and all fish and shellfish are great food sources of tyrosine. Eggs, milk, pulses, peanuts and almonds supply not only tyrosine, but also vitamin B12. For folic acid you should eat fortified-bran breakfast cereals, spinach, broccoli, lettuce and avocado. Milk, nuts and seeds supply magnesium in healthy doses.

38 Spice up your life

Too much salt in your diet can
cause bloating and fatigue, while
increasing your risk of high blood pressure.

You can't – and shouldn't – avoid salt
altogether in your diet, but you can take steps to
reduce your intake. Bear in mind that many food
labels list salt as sodium or sodium chloride.
Some foods claim to be 'reduced salt' or 'low salt',
but this can be confusing when the label talks in
terms of sodium. To find out how much salt is in
the food, multiply the sodium content figure by
2.5. Aim for less than 5 g (¼ oz) of salt a day.

Try to get out of the habit of adding salt to
your cooking, and avoid foods high in salt such
as cured and smoked meats, tinned meats,
salted nuts, sauces, ketchups, crisps and
crackers. Instead of adding salt to your food
when you cook, flavour it with herbs, spices,
lemon juice or ginger. Herbs and spices are full
of antioxidants and phyto-chemicals.
Antioxidants are used to help the body mop up
unhealthy free radicals formed by the oxygen we
breathe, and help to release energy from the

food we eat. If free radicals build up in our bodies they can cause damage, and they are also linked to many of the signs of ageing. Think of herbs and spices as being like extra compounds in high-grade fuel. They help your body engine use the carbohydrate fuel efficiently and reduce the build-up of deposits on moving engine parts. All this and they taste great, too.

Basil, chervil, dill, fennel and garlic work well with salads. Thyme, tarragon and parsley can really enhance the flavour of meat, fish, vegetables and potatoes. Have fun experimenting with spices or alternatives to salt to find out those you like best. You will gradually be able to adjust to a less salty diet and learn to appreciate the more subtle flavours of food that were once hidden by the overpowering taste of salt.

The more you wake your taste buds up and challenge them with new and exciting herbs, spices and flavours, the more alert you'll feel after eating. Try Indian, Thai or Chinese food, or opposing flavours like sweet and sour. If you go for Chinese food, make sure you skip the MSG (monosodium glutamate), which will have the opposite effect.

Boost energy with movement

Note: If you are overweight, have high blood pressure or a pre-existing medical condition, consult your doctor before beginning any exercise programme.

39 Get your 30 a day

When you're feeling run down it's hard to believe that exerting yourself actually gives you more energy, but here's how it works.

When you exercise regularly your muscles adapt and increase in size, boosting your metabolism (fat-burning) and stamina. Your heart and vascular system (which transports blood) also become more efficient, improving the delivery of energising oxygen that reaches your cells so you feel more awake. The more you exercise, the more efficient this process becomes and the more energy you have.

Exercise also increases your immunity and makes you feel good. And when you feel good, you have the energy to complete your daily tasks. Just 30 minutes' moderate to vigorous aerobic exercise has been shown to improve both mood and energy levels. Aerobic exercises like running or fast walking, done in the morning, will rev you up for several hours.

For optimum energy-boosting, try to get 30 minutes' cardiovascular exercise every day – that's exercise where you move continuously, such as jogging or brisk walking. Choose an activity you enjoy, as you are more likely to stick to it. You might enjoy walking or biking, swimming, dancing, gardening or ice-skating. It doesn't have to be an aerobic class. Start at a comfortable speed and gradually increase the intensity after 5 minutes. You should break into a light sweat and be slightly breathless, but not so breathless that you can't hold a conversation.

When you feel fit enough, why not sign up for a charity walk or join a sports team. When you have a specific goal or other people are relying on you, you're more likely to stick to your workouts.

40 Walk the talk

There are plenty of activities you can easily fit into your daily routine that will help to keep you fit and boost your energy levels.

Walk the talk: Buy a cordless phone and walk around the house when you're talking.

Increase your steps: Take the stairs instead of the lift, use the upstairs loo rather than the downstairs one, hide the remote controls and get up to switch your appliances on and off. Buy a pedometer to count your steps.

Out in the garden: Researchers at Kansas State University say gardening can strengthen limbs, help the cardiovascular system and develop flexibility.

Do it to music: Put on a lively CD and do your housework in time to it. You'll be working out without even knowing it.

Rediscover your sexual energy: Sex is a calorie burner and can be a good aerobic workout, too. It also releases feel-good hormones that increase your energy levels and put you in a good mood. So feel free to indulge yourself.

41 Break it down

According to a Stanford University research study, three 10-minute workout sessions (morning, lunch and evening) produce the same energising benefit as a solid 30-minute workout. So maybe a 10-minute jog in the morning, a 10-minute walk at lunch, and another 10-minute brisk walk at night might be easier for those of us who haven't got sufficient hours in the day.

Researchers at Northern Arizona State University also found that if you take as little as a 10-minute brisk walk a day, fatigue can disappear for up to two hours. This is because moving increases the flow of oxygen in your bloodstream and causes your brain to release mood-boosting chemicals. Not only will you feel more energised – you will also be burning calories.

A simple walk around the block can achieve all this, proving to those who feel too busy to exercise that simply increasing the time you already spend on certain activities – such as walking to work, dancing to your favourite music and walking your dog – is enough to build stamina and beat fatigue.

42 Sit up in front of the television

For the energy of strong muscles, endurance and flexibility, you need strength-training, flexibility and cardiovascular activity. Don't make the mistake of skipping strength-training and working only on your cardiovascular system. For stamina and endurance, you need muscle power.

Strength-training won't make your muscles look bulky and unattractive if done correctly – Marilyn Monroe used to lift weights. Clever strength exercises – lifting weights, yoga or light dumbbell work on your own at home – can reap great streamlining, energy-boosting rewards. If none of these appeals to you, find ways in your daily life to use your muscles more. Carry your shopping bags, lift your kids or do some squats, sit-ups and press-ups as you watch television.

Squats: Stand with your feet shoulder-width apart. Bend your knees and slowly start to sit down. Once your bottom is nearly in line with your knees, simply push up into a standing position, squeezing your bottom as you do. Do three sets of 10 repetitions; more if you feel able. Rest for a minute between sets.

Press-ups: Go down on your hands and knees and gently bend your elbows and straighten them again, keeping your back as straight as you can. If you have the muscle strength, assume the proper press-up position with your legs stretched out behind, balancing on the balls of your feet and your body parallel to the floor. Do three sets of 10 repetitions; more if you feel able. Rest for a minute between sets.

Sit-ups: Lie flat on the floor on your back with your knees bent and feet flat on the floor. Place your hands lightly behind your head. Using your abdominals, lift your shoulders a few inches off the floor, pause briefly and return to your starting position. Complete three sets of ten repetitions; more if you feel up to it. Rest for a minute between sets. If you don't think you have time, all of these simple toning exercises can be done while you watch your favourite soap or TV programme.

43 Train Swedish style

Are you stuck in an exercise rut? Running the same number of miles a week? Swimming the same number of lengths? When muscles get used to an exercise pattern, they begin to adapt. Your body gets used to a particular type of exercise and burns fewer calories doing it. To keep your calorie burn, energy and motivation high, mix your workouts. Combine walking with cycling, jogging with swimming, or stair-climbing with aerobics, and so on.

Try to vary the intensity of your workout, too. In Sweden the routine is taken out of exercise by a training method known as 'fartlek'. This type of training can increase both your fitness and your energy levels.

Go as fast as you can for as long as you feel comfortable; then slow down. When the urge hits, do sit-ups and press-ups – whatever it is that keeps you moving and having fun, even if it means skipping your way through 30 minutes of your workout. If you are having fun, you are more likely to be motivated to finish your workout.

44 Swing in the morning

Any form of exercise in the morning boosts your circulation and sends a signal to your brain that it's time to wake up and kick into gear. If you haven't got time to work out, the following yoga exercise will help energise you first thing.

Stand with your feet hip-distance apart and swing your arms by your sides. Turn your upper body from side to side, slowly swinging your arms so that they gently slap against your body. Each time you turn, look over the shoulder you are swinging towards and lift the opposite heel. Inhale through your nose as you turn to the front and exhale through your mouth as you swing to the side. Do this for at least 2 minutes. The gentle swinging motion is both relaxing and energising at the same time and can be done whenever you feel stressed or drowsy.

45 Straighten up

Having good posture affects not only how confident you look to others; it also provides you with many other health benefits. Primarily, these health benefits occur because when your posture is correct, your muscles, organs, joints and bones are all where they're supposed to be. If you stand or sit with an incorrect posture, unnecessary energy-draining strain is inevitable.

Poor posture can come from many sources, including incorrect sitting and standing habits, obesity, pregnancy, an improperly arranged work environment, not enough flexibility and weak muscles. Signs that you may have poor posture include: slouching and hunching your shoulders over, holding your head and neck forward and/or down, carrying a heavy bag or backpack on one side of your body, holding a phone receiver between your neck and shoulder, and slumping forward while seated.

Want to check your posture? Stand with your back to a wall. If your shoulders, bottom and the back of your head are all touching the wall, then your posture is correct.

Good posture tips while sitting

✔ Keep both feet flat on the floor (if your feet cannot reach the floor, adjust the chair or use a footrest).

✔ Align your back with the back of the chair. Don't slouch or lean forward.

✔ Adjust the chair so your knees are even with your hips, or slightly higher, and your arms are at a 75–90° angle at the elbows.

✔ Keep your shoulders straight.

✔ Get up often and stretch.

Good posture tips while standing

✔ Keep your weight on the balls of your feet, not your heels.

✔ Let your arms hang naturally by your side.

✔ Keep your feet about shoulder-width apart.

✔ Don't lock your knees.

✔ Keep your head level and in line with your neck and spine, not pushed forward.

✔ Keep your shoulders upright and stand up straight.

46 Deskersize

If your job is desk-bound there
are plenty of things you can do
to keep fit and energetic. As well
as making sure you get up and have a stretch or
a short walk every half an hour or so, try some of
the following exercises today:

Calf stretch: Remove your shoes and place
your feet flat on the floor with your knees slightly
apart. Bring your toes up towards the front of
your legs while keeping your heels on the floor.
This will help iron out kinks in your calves.

60-second aerobics: While seated, pump
both arms over your head for 30 seconds, then
rapidly tap your feet on the floor, football-drill
style, for 30 seconds. Repeat 3–5 times.

Body lift: Place your hands on the arms of
your chair and lift yourself up slightly. Repeat.

Buttock squeeze: Tighten and squeeze your
buttocks, hold for 5 to 10 seconds, and release.
Repeat 6 to 8 times. Really concentrate on the
'squeeze' for the best results.

Straight and narrow: Sit up straight in
your chair.

47 Dance, rock and growl

Dancing is a great energiser. Sadly many of us feel too self-conscious to really let go. If this is the case, try dancing at home when no one is looking, or – if you are in company – closing your eyes.

Put on some rock, disco, rhythm and blues or any kind of music that gets your feet tapping and move to the music, releasing your body's energy. If there is no opportunity to dance, try rocking. Rocking has been shown to enhance the nervous and musculature systems. As you rock, your stomach, back and thigh muscles are gently stimulated, as is the fluid of your inner ear, which some studies have shown can increase alertness. A rocking chair is great but, if you haven't got one on standby, swaying gently from side to side or forward and back as you stand or sit can be equally beneficial.

Another great energy release if you don't feel like dancing or rocking is to move the muscles of your face. During the day a lot of tension can build up in our faces, especially around the eyes. Make faces or growl as hard as you can to release the tension in your face.

48 Fidget

The amount of small movements you make can be the difference between fit and fat. So if you're not a fidget, teach yourself to be one. When you're doing nothing in particular, try drumming your fingers, changing position, twirling your pen, pacing up and down, and tapping your fingers and feet.

This is especially important if you have to sit in one spot for long periods of time – such as at your desk, or on a plane or train. In these situations blood gets drawn from your brain and heart and pools in your legs; this can make you feel sluggish and tired. The more you fidget, the more you keep the blood pumping around your body and ensure that your energy levels are up. So don't sit for long periods; get up and walk around or, at the very least, move your legs or change the position you sit in. A good stretch or yawn or shoulder roll to release tension will also help.

49 Do the twist

Twisting the body boosts energy because it releases tension along the spine and stimulates digestion. Sit on a chair or cross-legged on the floor and extend your arms to the side. From this position, gently turn to your right and place your left hand on your right thigh or knee, depending on whether you are sitting on a chair or the floor, while bringing your right hand up behind your back. Feel each vertebra moving, and be gentle with your neck. Take several breaths, twisting slightly more each time you breathe out. Release the twist on an exhale and repeat on the other side. You can also do this exercise in a standing position, but whether you sit or stand, to avoid the risk of back injury make sure your movements are slow and controlled.

50 Kickstart with a brush

Skin brushing – also called dry body brushing – is a simple, invigorating technique that stimulates blood and lymph flow, exfoliates the skin, encourages new cell growth and can make you feel great.

To brush your skin, start at your feet and sweep up the legs in long, light, brisk movements. All skin-brushing movements should be towards the heart, to encourage the return of blood and encourage lymphatic flow.

Brush your abdomen with a circular motion. Body brushes should take about 3 to 5 minutes, depending on how many strokes you give each spot. Don't be too rough. Over-brushing causes the skin to turn red and become irritated. The best time to body brush is first thing in the morning, when the increased blood flow will help wake you up, or before you take a shower.

Skin brushes are fairly inexpensive and readily available at most chemists and supermarkets.

51 Supercharge your life

Studies have shown that when you move faster, your metabolism speeds up. Acting energetically can therefore make you feel more energetic.

We think we act because of the way we feel, but often we feel because of the way we act. The idea is to trick yourself into feeling energetic by moving more quickly, pacing while you talk on the phone, putting more energy into your voice, and so on. It's a simple energy-boosting strategy that is surprisingly effective. So the next time you feel your energy take a nose-dive, even if you don't feel energetic try acting energetically by moving, working or talking faster than normal. You can also apply this technique when your mood or motivation to do something is low. Simply pretend you are excited. More often than not this tricks your brain and you start feeling excited.

52 Five energising stretches

Before and after a workout it is important to warm up and cool down your muscles by gently stretching them. Stretching not only improves your flexibility and prevents the risk of injury; it's a great way to release tension and re-energise.

To give your body and mind a wake-up call, hold the following stretches for 20 to 30 seconds with deep breathing throughout.

Neck and shoulders: Stand tall. Lace your fingers behind your head as if you were lying back. Take a deep breath. Exhale and slowly tuck your chin into your chest and press your head down and forward. Inhale as you lift to the starting position.

Back: Sit on the edge of a chair with your feet hip-distance apart and flat on the floor. Take a deep breath and tuck your chin into your chest. With your arms by your side, slowly roll forwards until your chest is resting on your thighs and you are folded in half. Breathe deeply and, as you exhale, uncurl your back into a straight-up position.

Legs: Sit on the edge of a seat with your feet flat on the floor. Extend your right leg straight in front of you and flex your toes towards the ceiling. Relax and place both hands on your left thigh, take a deep breath and lean forward as you exhale. Feel the stretch in the back of your right leg. Repeat on the other side.

Arms: In a standing position, straighten your right arm and gently place it across your body at shoulder height. Hug your right upper arm with your left hand and press it against your body. Breathe deeply, rest and change sides to repeat.

Whole body: Lie on your back with your legs together and extend your arms over your head, in line with your shoulders. Keep your head in line with your spine. Pull your tummy in tightly and press your lower back firmly to the floor. Take a deep breath in and, as you breathe out, extend both your arms and legs as far away from your body as you can. Breathing normally, hold the stretch for a count of 10 and relax. You can also do this exercise standing up; simply stretch as far as you can on the balls of your feet towards the ceiling and relax.

Boost energy naturally

53 Breathing for energy

Proper breathing is perhaps the easiest and most powerful way to boost your energy. It results in better digestion and circulation, more stable heart rate, decreased stress and more restful sleep. Most of us don't think that much about it and fall into the habit of breathing shallowly and rapidly, especially when we feel stressed or tense. Breathing in this way can make you feel tired and muzzy-headed; you are also likely to yawn more in order to increase your oxygen intake.

Learning how to breathe correctly from the diaphragm is simple. Keep your hand on your abdomen and, when you breathe in, make the abdomen rise. You will find that your abdomen rises and falls but your upper chest stays still.

54 Refresh with alternate-nostril breathing

There are a number of simple breathing techniques to help you maximise your intake of energising oxygen, especially when you're under stress. The quickest way to recharge is to get more oxygen into your body by taking deep breaths.

Try this simple exercise. For 5 minutes twice a day, breathe in to a count of 4, then out to a count of 8, making a 'whoosh' sound.

Another yoga breathing exercise that can help release tension is called alternate-nostril breathing.

Rest the thumb of your right hand lightly against your right nostril while breathing in to a count of 4 through your left nostril.

Close both nostrils to a count of 4 by keeping your thumb in position and using the little finger of your right hand to close your left nostril.

Remove your thumb and breathe out through your right nostril to a count of 4.

Pause for a moment before completing the cycle by breathing in through the right nostril first.

55 Light up

Light – in particular strong light, such as sunlight – is the most powerful regulator of our biological clock, which influences when we feel sleepy or alert. Bright sunlight (or any bright light) tells your body's natural biological clock that it's time to wake up; that same clock will then be set to tell your body it's time to go to sleep about 14–16 hours later.

The amount of exposure you get to light during the day may interfere with the quality of your sleep and how alert you feel during the day. Studies have shown there is a link between light exposure and sleep. This is because higher light levels during the day help regulate the biological clock, which coordinates a number of bodily functions including the secretion of melatonin, an important factor in well-balanced sleeping patterns. So whether you are a lark who likes to rise and go to bed early, or an owl who likes to get up and go to bed later – or even a humming-bird somewhere in between – make sure that at some point in the day you go outside and expose yourself to the energy-boosting power of daylight. This is especially important during the winter months when you may start and leave work in darkness. Being cooped up in the house or office all day will drain your energy. Research has shown that people need at least 30 minutes of natural sunlight a day to keep their brain producing feel-good hormones. If you wear glasses or contact lenses try taking them off, but always be careful to avoid looking directly at the sun.

If you are a night owl and want to have more energy in the morning, expose yourself to at least 15 minutes of bright light soon after waking. Without your glasses, sunglasses or contact lenses, go outside and get some daylight. Don't look directly at the sun.

Being outside in natural light will gradually cause your period of night-time sleep to occur earlier. Similarly, a morning lark who doesn't want to be accused of being a 'party pooper' should get bright light exposure before sleeping. Artificial sun boxes are made for this purpose.

56 Stay cool

If you spend a lot of time
indoors with the central heating
on, not only are you depriving
yourself of the energising effects of
oxygen but you are also more likely to become
dehydrated, which is another energy-drainer.
This is because warm air holds more moisture
than cold air, so if you heat up the air without
adding moisture, it sucks moisture out of your
skin to compensate. You are also more likely to
get headaches and to find it hard to concentrate.

Try turning the heating down and wearing
more clothing, and see if it makes a difference to
your energy levels. If central heating is a must,
then it is advisable to humidify the air. Plug-in
humidifiers are available in the shops to do this,
or small magnetic pots can be bought fairly
cheaply that you just fill with water and stick to
the radiator. Houseplants can help a little, too.

57 Power down

Electrical sensitivity – when electrical currents interfere with your body's natural rhythms – has been blamed for unexplained skin and eye problems, sleep problems and fatigue, problems thinking, difficulty concentrating and headaches.

Cordless phones may be the worst culprits as we tend to keep them beside the bed, where we receive electrical waves from the base. Other risk factors include using the hairdryer for more than 10 minutes, keeping a digital clock by the bed, and sitting too close and too long in front of a computer screen.

To reduce your risk, switch to an analogue battery-operated clock and unplug electrical goods before you go to bed. Keep your wireless network router in a different room to your study or bedroom, and switch off your computer rather than using a screensaver. If you're working in front of a computer screen for long periods at a time, make sure you take a few minutes' break every half hour or so; do some stretching, deep breathing and look far away into the distance to refocus your eyes.

58 Pavement sense

If you live or work in the city or near a busy road, you increase your exposure to energy-draining carbon monoxide fumes and toxins.

One of the best ways to reduce your exposure to air pollution is to avoid walking along busy streets and thoroughfares. Instead, choose side streets and parks. Carefully selecting your route will have a dramatic effect because pollution levels can fall by a factor of 10 just by moving a few metres away from the main source of the pollution – exhaust fumes. Even being one street away makes a massive difference, as high pollution levels are generally restricted to fairly small areas within a city. Also try to avoid walking down 'street canyons' (where tall buildings hug tightly to the sides of streets, creating valleys in which pollutants build up), don't walk behind smokers, and walk on the windward side of the street where exposure to pollutants can be 50 per cent less than on the leeward side.

When you're crossing a road, stand well back from the kerb while you wait for the lights to change or for a gap in the traffic. Every metre really does count when you are in close proximity to traffic, so do all you can to avoid getting stuck for too long on a central reservation. As the traffic moves off from a standstill, the fumes can dissipate in just a few seconds, particularly if the wind is up; holding your breath during this momentary period can make a difference, silly as it might sound.

Also, don't dawdle: cross the road as quickly as possible. And once you're over, continue along the pavement as far away from the kerb as possible. Remember, the more distance you put between yourself and traffic, the less likely you are to breath in unwanted and energy-draining fumes and toxins.

59 What a shower!

If your morning routine involves a hot shower immediately after waking, this may be a contributing factor towards mid-morning fatigue. Hot showers raise your body temperature and encourage the production of sleep hormones a few hours later.

The ideal water temperature for a shower is 35°C (95°F). This temperature makes the water feel pleasant and does not overstrain your circulatory system. If you want to feel even more refreshed and invigorated, take a cooler shower.

A shower that is too hot can make your body feel tired, but if you can't give up your hot morning shower, turn the cold water on for the last 2 minutes. The alternating temperature causes your blood vessels to open and contract, increasing your circulation, which in turn stimulates your digestion, your elimination and your overall energy levels. The different temperatures also mimic the fluctuating air temperatures outside. If you can get used to the hot/cold shower technique, maybe the day-to-day changes in the weather won't be so draining.

60 See green

To reduce your risk of exposure to energy-draining environmental toxins, try to take a stroll in a park or green place at least once a day.

Trees give out energising oxygen. A number of studies have shown that people have more energy and a better attention span after spending time close to nature or simply playing a round of golf. The research shows that you don't even need to be out for long; as little as 20 minutes in a place that is even slightly green is far better than 20 minutes indoors.

Try to get a nature boost in as many different ways as you can. Go outside, sit by the window, have lunch in the park or buy yourself a goldfish! It's also a good idea to have plants in your home and workplace. A living, breathing green plant can take in carbon monoxide and give off energising oxygen to keep your mind alert and your energy levels high. NASA research has shown that the following plants can extract fumes, chemicals and smoke from the air: peace lilies, dwarf banana plants, spider plants, weeping figs, geraniums and chrysanthemums.

61 Stimulating smells

Each of us has a secret source of energy which you can't see but which can boost your energy, mood and motivation without you even knowing it. It's a smell. Not just any smell, but a particular smell that invigorates you. It's different for everyone. For some it's apples, for others peppermint, leather or roasted chestnuts.

The fact that odours can boost energy isn't news to people familiar with the basics of aromatherapy. We've heard for years about the effects smells have on our brains and bodies. Grapefruit, for example, can be used to refresh and revive. In Japan there's a company that pipes in scented air to pep up employees. In the morning, cedar and cypress wake them up. In the afternoon, citrus stimulates their senses.

Filling a room with the right scents at the right times can be an energy boost. Your sense of smell is, after all, one of the most powerful of your senses – the one that can send the most vivid messages to your brain and evoke the most vivid images. It's best to avoid the overpowering smells and chemicals used in artificial air fresheners and to use the natural scents of essential oils instead. Aromatherapists will often recommend lavender, rosemary, geranium, peppermint, ginger, grapefruit, lemon and orange essential oils for boosting energy, but it is best to experiment and find what works well for you.

Essential oils are typically very strong and are not made to be placed directly on the skin. To use them as massage oil, mix a few drops with 1 or 2 tsp of a carrier oil (a neutral-smelling oil that is good for skin and massage, such as sweet almond, sunflower or jojoba oil). Another method for using essential oils is in an oil burner or diffuser. A few drops of oil can be enough to fill the room with a great smell, helping you relax as soon as you step in the door. Alternatively, you could add a few drops to a handkerchief and inhale when you feel your energy levels take a nose-dive.

62 Open a window

Inadequate ventilation means you aren't getting the energy-boosting benefits of oxygen. It also increases the level of pollutants and emissions that you breathe, which in turn puts you at a higher risk of poor health, including respiratory problems, headaches and fatigue.

Open a window if you can, but if this isn't an option, buy an ionizer. Exhaust fumes from cars, trucks and buses, emission from factories, cigarette smoke, dust, soot and electromagnetic pollution all combine to create a harmful mixture of positive ions, and reduces the proportion of beneficial negative ions in our surroundings. This gradually affects our lungs, can ruin our health and cause general lethargy, fatigue and depression.

63 Detox your home

Stoves, heaters and dryers that burn fuel of any kind may generate energy-draining carbon monoxide and nitrogen dioxide. If the appliance is improperly maintained or ventilated, carbon monoxide poisoning can occur. Chronic low-grade exposure may cause subtle deterioration in mental function, and also hearing loss. Sometimes the first signs of carbon monoxide toxicity in the home are morning headache, dizziness and having difficulty concentrating.

The solution is simple but very important: if you haven't got one already, buy a carbon monoxide detector immediately. It could save your life. And when you have bought a carbon monoxide detector be sure to check the batteries regularly.

· ·

Improving the air quality in your home will help you breathe better and reduce your risk of fatigue and headaches caused by pollutants that can trigger energy-draining allergies. For better breathing, try the following:

Change your shower curtain. Mould doesn't just do damage to your house but also to your body; symptoms include headaches, poor concentration, rashes and fatigue. Shower curtains make an especially good home in which mould can grow, so you should replace your shower curtain if it has a large amount of mould on it. If the mould is minimal, you can remove the shower curtain, scrub it with a household cleaner and rinse before re-hanging.

Dust and vacuum as much as you can. Use a damp cloth when dusting to capture the dust. Wear a dust mask to prevent inhalation of dust particles. Keep small objects, such as knick-knacks, in drawers or closed cabinets to minimise the chore of dusting.

When oil is heated, bubbles are formed which burst into the air, releasing noxious irritants.

Be aware of vapours and use extractor fans when cooking.

Curtains are major dust-magnets. If feasible, replace curtains with shades or blinds made of plastic or other washable materials to allow for easy cleaning. If you must use curtains, wash them regularly.

Kerosene and space heaters produce nitrogen dioxide which can irritate your eyes, nose and throat, and cause difficulty in your breathing. Avoid using them.

Carpets generate a lot of dust. If you have old carpet, consider replacing it with another type of flooring and using throw rugs that can be laundered.

Air out your dry-cleaning. The cleaning fluids used to clean your clothes could be making you tired, so air (preferably outside) new clothes and clothes that have been dry-cleaned. When the chemical smell has gone it means that the solvents have evaporated.

65 Kick off your shoes

Remove your shoes when you get back home. In homes where people do not routinely remove their shoes, the house dust is often loaded with lead and other energy-draining environmental toxins which are brought in from outdoors. Carpeting holds up to a hundred times the amount of dust as bare flooring; the deeper the pile, the harder it is to remove the dust.

A great deal of attention has been focused on old, lead-based paint that peels and flakes from walls and ceilings as a source of low-level lead exposure. What is less well known is that much roadside soil is still poisoned with lead deposited by petrol fumes emitted before the ban on leaded petroleum additives, and that the soil around houses becomes contaminated with lead during new home construction or home renovation. This lead is brought into the house on your shoes, increasing the lead levels in air and dust.

66 Tidy up

When your energy is low, the last thing you might want to do is have a tidy up – but cleaning or tidying can be a fantastic energy boost. An untidy, cluttered house can drain you of energy; the simple act of cleaning and tidying helps you create order out of chaos, which in itself is a great feeling.

Think about how you feel when you walk into someone else's space that's cluttered full of unnecessary junk. Compare that with how it feels to walk into a light, spacious, airy room. The space gives a sense of possibility and lightness, as well as the opportunity to think clearly, express yourself openly and be altogether more expansive.

You don't need to go overboard and give your entire house a full spring clean. Simply choose one room in your house, put on some music and tidy that room up. Throw out or give away what you don't need any more. Pay special attention to piles of paper and other clutter, because mounds of clutter can drain your energy and weigh you down.

67 Look ahead

A rushed, disorganised morning can drain your energy before the day has even started. Before you go to bed tonight, make sure you get everything organised for tomorrow morning. Check the weather forecast for the morning and put your clothes, watch, shoes, bag and jewellery out on a chair ready for when you wake up. Then in the morning you can give your body and mind time to wake up without worrying about what you need to wear or what you need to bring with you. With your clothes laid out and your day scheduled you can wake up and prepare for your day ahead in a calm state of mind so that when your day swings into action you have the energy you need to enjoy it.

68 Refreshing sounds

Daily exposure to unwanted, disruptive noises such as traffic, airplanes, car alarms, mobile phones, raised voices and road repairs can drain your energy without you even realising it. It's impossible to switch off the surrounding noise when you are outside your home, so as compensation you need to make sure that you enjoy the mood-enhancing benefits of sound whenever you can.

Music is a great healer and energiser when you are feeling low. Don't be afraid to expand your music collection. Discovering a new musical style or artist can bring you an enormous amount of pleasure. Don't feel, though, that music is the only way to boost your mood or induce a sense of calm – the sound of silence can be the most refreshing sound in the world. Wind chimes can also create a magical and exciting effect, as can the sound of running water from a water feature in your house or garden.

69 Make your mind up

Procrastination, or putting things off, drains you of purposeful energy. Instead of taking determined decisions and actions, you end up fretting over all the things you haven't done or the things that you feel you should do. You will use up most of your energy simply in justifying putting things off until another day and feeling bad about your indecisiveness and inactivity. If you tend to procrastinate, making your mind up about something will give you an instant energy boost. It will remind you that you are in control of your life.

Weigh up all the pros and cons, think carefully about what you want and then make a decision, even if that decision is not to make a decision. If you find it hard to move beyond worry and indecision, remind yourself that taking action when faced with dilemmas can be far less stressful than feeling anxious about them. If your solution or decision didn't work, don't torture yourself with anxiety. Try to understand why it didn't work or where you went wrong, and use that knowledge to seek another solution.

70 Get time on your side

You can give your energy a significant boost simply by being more organised. Try to plan ahead as much as you can: prepare the night before, write a shopping list ahead of going to the supermarket so you don't forget what you need, and so on. Writing a daily schedule will also help.

Take a look at your present routine, what your priorities and your goals are, then organise your day according to these priorities and goals. Tackle the hardest jobs in the morning when you have the most energy, and avoid putting things off until the last minute. If at all possible delegate some of your tasks; it's exhausting trying to do everything yourself.

In order to manage your time effectively you need to devise a system that meets your needs but is also flexible. If you think you haven't got time to sit down and consider your schedule, remind yourself that time management is an investment that always pays off. You will feel calmer and more in control of your life, better prepared and, above all, more energetic.

71 Paint the walls orange

In physics, colours correspond to electromagnetic frequencies. There is no doubt that colours affect your energy levels. Many of us associate colours with emotions and concepts: red suggests passion, black conjures up intensity, yellow means youth, and so on. The most stimulating colours are often those that correspond to the natural world, for example sky blue and deep green.

Changing the colour in your living room or office can boost your energy by highlighting your colour responses. Orange, pale red, green and yellow tend to be the colours most often associated with energy – but before you redecorate, choose a colour that gives you a boost. You don't have to paint the whole room; simply painting the wall behind your desk can help enliven your senses. And if painting isn't an option, add a splash of colour into your environment with posters, pictures or fabrics.

72 Just say 'Omm'!

The purpose of meditation isn't to boost energy, but that can certainly be one of its many benefits. This is because when you meditate your heart rate and breathing slow down, your blood pressure normalises, you use oxygen more efficiently, your adrenal glands produce less of the stress hormone cortisol, your mind clears and your creativity and concentration improve.

Meditation involves sitting in a relaxed position and clearing your mind. You may focus on a sound, such as 'Omm', on your own breathing, or on nothing at all. When distracting thoughts arise, notice them and let them go.

Spiritual masters say that the purpose of meditation is simply to be. This can be an incredibly hard concept to grasp when you have a long list of to-dos demanding your energy and time. But learning to quiet your mind and body will boost your mental and physical energy, helping you to feel more in control when things don't go as planned.

73 Creative cloud-spotting

If meditation isn't your thing, there are many other ways to re-energise by turning inward. You can doodle, listen to music without words, daydream or do whatever allows you to tune out, refresh your mind and tap into your intuition. Intuition and flashes of insight can give you an incredible energy boost; suddenly the solution to a problem or the way forward becomes clear. Intuition isn't always easy to recognise but it tends to appear when you let your mind wander and give your imagination free rein.

To tap into your intuitive energy and latent creativity, go outside or look out of a window and stare at the clouds in the sky. Make sure you don't stare intently at the clouds, just look at them vaguely as if you were daydreaming. If it's a sunny day make sure that you don't look directly at the sun. Keep looking at the clouds and see what shapes appear. Notice what images you can identify and ask yourself what these images mean to you.

74 On your toes

According to reflexologists,
the tensions and stresses in
your body are mirrored in and
released in the soles of your feet.
The toes correspond to your head and face,
the heel to your lower back, the arch to your
digestive organs.

Even if you are sceptical about the benefits
of reflexology, there is no doubt that a foot
massage feels great, so visit a reflexologist if
you want to give your body and mind a lift.
Alternatively you can stretch your feet and toes
any time you like. Kick off your shoes and give
your feet a gentle rub. Then roll your ankles;
stretch and separate your toes; press down
through the balls of your feet, and lift your toes
and the balls of your feet off the floor.

75 Revive with yoga

Studies have found that yoga, the 5,000-year-old Hindu system of exercises, improves attention, memory, endurance and concentration.

To whet your appetite for yoga, one really effective way to beat fatigue is to try a yoga pose known as the 'Standing Stretch'. Stand in the correct posture – that is, with your toes pointing forward, your knees relaxed and your feet at hip-width apart. Ensure your weight is balanced evenly between the ball and the heel of your foot. Interlace your thumbs and stretch your hands up above your head while keeping your arms against your ears – and stretch upwards from the lumbar area of your lower back. Keeping your breath even throughout, now slowly release your arms down in front of you. Tuck your chin into your chest bone and gently lower yourself down, vertebra by vertebra, keeping your arms hanging loosely and then just hang from the waist. This position encourages the blood flow to your head and is a real winner when you need to energise yourself. After 1 minute, slowly bring yourself back up into a standing position. Repeat this whole procedure 3 times.

76 Go with the flow

Energy medicine techniques such as acupuncture, Reiki and therapeutic touch are based on the understanding that your body has an energy flow running through it and that health problems are caused by blockages or excesses in this flow. Treatment aims to free up blocked energy in the body so that healing can occur.

In Traditional Chinese Medicine, this energy flow is called *Qi* (chi). For acupuncture, tiny needles are used to stimulate chi along 14 body meridians, or energy pathways. There are a number of studies to suggest that something happens along these pathways that can affect our health and energy levels.

Acupuncture has been found to be effective in treating many disorders, including fatigue. If you want to give it a try, make sure you consult an accredited acupuncturist.

If the thought of needles going into your body doesn't appeal, you could always try acupressure, which is based on the same principles as acupuncture but uses hand or finger pressure instead of needles.

77 Clear as crystal

Crystals, like everything else on this planet, are made of energy, store energy and conduct energy. They have been used in healing by many different cultures and civilizations for many thousands of years. The ancient Egyptians, for example, would grind down crystals and drink them for their healing properties.

Each crystal holds and conducts its own frequency of energy (due to the speed at which the energy vibrates). This energy is known by science as electromagnetic energy. The different energy frequencies of different crystals are thought to influence different parts of our mind and body. Turquoise, for example, is thought to help balance and regulate energy. Ruby is thought to encourage passion for life. Quartz is thought to restore energy and optimism. To give it a try, you may want to place crystals in your office or home, or wear them as jewellery. If nothing else, they will add a splash of colour and sparkle to your life.

78 Motivating massage

Nothing feels quite as good or is quite as energising as a massage. If you don't want to book one, ask your partner or a friend to give you a 5-minute massage to loosen your neck and shoulders, because the more tense your neck and shoulders are, the more likely you are to feel tense and tired. You could also give your shoulders an energising DIY massage.

To massage tense shoulders, stroke your right shoulder with your left hand. Then, starting at the base of your skull, stroke down the side of your neck, over your shoulder and down your arm to the elbow. Glide back to your neck and repeat at least 3 times. Then do the other side.

Apply circular pressure with your fingertips on either side of your spine. Work up your neck and around the base of your skull. Then knead each shoulder, squeezing and releasing the flesh on your shoulders and at the top of your arms.

Loosely clench your left hand into a fist and gently pound your right shoulder. Keep your wrist flexible.

79 Achieve optimum balance

When life is busy or the pressure mounts it is very easy to forget that the key to health and energy is *balance*.

So if you have been working really hard you need to make sure that you find time to refresh your energy and motivation. It doesn't matter how you choose to do this; some people like to meditate, while others like to party. It all depends on the kind of person you are, but any of the following are highly recommended:

✔ soak in an aromatherapy bath
✔ have an early night
✔ take a long walk in the fresh air, perhaps along a beach
✔ go to the movies
✔ enjoy a massage
✔ get your hair done
✔ have fun with your family
✔ phone a friend.

The main thing is that you find ways to ensure you have enough time to recharge your batteries.

It's also extremely important that you don't feel guilty about taking time out for yourself.

80 5-minute stress-management techniques

Stress overload is a huge energy-drainer, so it is essential to learn how to manage stress effectively before it wears you down physically and emotionally. It is important to take some time out to regain an element of control. Here are some stress-management techniques that you can experiment with in just 5 minutes a day!

Greeting people warmly, especially in the morning, is important to manage stress. You wonder why? Have you ever noticed how some people start the day grumpy? It is almost as if they have decided that they will be stressed out that day. When you greet someone warmly in the morning, it says you have decided that you will start a great day.

Take a few moments to close your eyes, take a deep breath and mentally consider various parts of your body in turn, from your feet upwards. Think about how each part feels at this particular moment – is it comfortable or tense? Concentrate particularly on your neck, jaw, face, forehead and abdomen. If they seem tense, allow them to relax one by one – feel the tension flowing away.

Concentrate on your breathing – breathe deeply in through your nose, then out slowly through your mouth. Make sure that your stomach area participates in the breathing process; this allows the full capacity of your lungs to be used.

Imagine that you are actually somebody else. It can be helpful if that person is someone you admire; this may be someone in your family, a film star or respected friend. Try to see the stressed 'you' from this other person's viewpoint – what would they consider to be important? How would they cope with the stresses with which you are faced?

Remember what you can and can't control. Don't get stressed trying to control people, because this is a hopeless task. You can't control the way other people think or behave; you can only control your attitude towards them. Every day ask yourself: What (or whom) do I need to give up trying to control so that I can have more energy for the things I can influence?

Take off your watch: watches are often a source of unnecessary and unhealthy stress. The next time you have a day off, try to go for a morning or afternoon without your watch on so you can appreciate what you are doing instead of how long it takes you to do it.

Set aside a few moments to decide for yourself which things are important, and which are just distractions. Decide which things you are going to do today, and which things you are not going to do today.

Create a habit of reviewing the positive that has happened throughout the day. Instead of crashing in front of the television when you reach home, spend 5 to 10 minutes reviewing what positive things have happened today. It can be as simple as someone holding a door open for you or catching your favourite piece of music on the radio; whatever it is, make sure you spend time focusing on it.

Acknowledge that stress can be good and make stress your friend! Based on the body's natural fight-or-flight response, that burst of energy can enhance your performance at the right moment.

Boost energy with supplements

• •

> **Note:** Large amounts of any herb or dietary supplement can be toxic and should only be taken under the guidance of a doctor or a qualified nutritional consultant or herbalist. If you are on any medication, have high blood pressure or diabetes, are pregnant or hoping to be, you should take herbs and supplements only under professional guidance.

If you decide to take supplements, do remember that they are what their name suggests – supplementary to your usual diet. They are *never* a substitute for a healthy, well-balanced diet. However, if you combine healthy eating with carefully chosen supplements you will optimise your chances of good health.

81 The energy vitamin

The energy-boosting benefits of vitamin C go far beyond its immune system potency. Along with a host of other benefits, vitamin C makes a chemical in your body called carnitine, which is needed by your muscles to burn energy. Vitamin C is essential if you want to turn the clock back. As an antioxidant, it protects your skin from environmental damage, prevents age spots and speeds up cell renewal for a more youthful glow. It also boosts collagen production, which means fewer wrinkles. When you are low in vitamin C this will show up as lethargy and fatigue.

Major sources of vitamin C are oranges and vegetables such as broccoli. Most of us simply don't get enough vitamin C a day. As most multivitamins and minerals don't contain enough vitamin C, supplementing separately may be one way to get your zing back. Most nutritionists recommend supplementing with 1,000 mg daily.

82 Get your multivitamin and mineral boost

A healthy diet is the basis for healthy energy levels, but because it isn't always easy to get all the nutrients you need for optimum health in your diet, taking supplements may be extremely beneficial. Even if you eat all the 'right foods', modern agricultural and production processes remove much of the nutritional value. For example, almost 80 per cent of zinc, a vital mineral for energy production, is removed from wheat during the milling process to ensure that bread has a longer shelf life.

The term 'supplement' covers a broad range of vitamins, minerals and plant extracts that should be taken to complement – not replace – a healthy, balanced diet. The most popular supplement is the multivitamin and mineral that most nutritionists regard as a good insurance policy and which can be taken over the long term.

To maximise your energy potential you can't afford to be deficient in any of the essential vitamins and minerals, so on top of a healthy diet you should consider taking a multivitamin and mineral supplement every day.

Supplements are best taken in the morning immediately after breakfast. If you combine them with other energy-boosting strategies – such as stress management and eating a balance of fresh vegetables and fruit, wholegrains, legumes, oily fish and nuts and seeds – you may be able to leave fatigue behind.

A number of vitamins and minerals help us to turn food into energy. You need them in varying amounts to feel your best during the day. Make sure that your multivitamin and mineral combination contains vitamins A, C and the B complex, as well as calcium, chromium, copper, iron, manganese, magnesium, selenium and zinc. You are also better off paying for quality supplements from reputable companies which, if asked, can supply you with independent analysis of their products. It's better to have half a quality tablet a day than the full dose of a mediocre one.

83 B complex, high strength

When it comes to energy boosting, studies have shown that the B complex vitamins – thiamine, riboflavin, niacin, B6, B12, folic acid, pantothenic acid and biotin – are most often linked to optimum mental and physical performance.

B vitamins help turn carbohydrates into the glucose energy that fuels your cells, muscles and brain. Each of them works in a slightly different way. Vitamin B3, for example, which is found in eggs, brewer's yeast, nuts, sunflower seeds, wholegrains and fish, helps release the energy from protein, carbohydrates and fats. It is needed to metabolise toxins and to form red blood cells and hormones. It also promotes a healthy digestive system, central nervous system and skin. Vitamin B5, found in eggs, nuts and wholegrains, is needed for the conversion of carbohydrates to energy. Vitamin B6, found in avocados, bananas, fish, meat, nuts, seeds and wholegrains, helps form neurotransmitters, the nerve chemicals that send messages to the brain. Vitamin B12, found in cheese, eggs, fish, lean meat and yoghurt, makes red blood cells that contain iron-rich haemoglobin and deliver energising oxygen to our cells. Folate or folic acid, found in leafy green vegetables, soya and wholegrains, works with vitamin B12 and makes amino acids, the building blocks of life-sustaining protein.

If you aren't getting enough B vitamins in your diet it will increase your risk of fatigue. As you get older you also need more B vitamins because over the years our bodies absorb less vitamin B12 even if we eat foods rich in it. Vegetarians can also often be at risk of vitamin B deficiency. Symptoms of B12 deficiency include headaches and fatigue.

The B vitamins work together like a team, so to supplement it is best to take a high-strength vitamin B complex tablet every day containing the whole range of B vitamins.

Note: If you are already taking a quality multivitamin and mineral, you may not need to take a vitamin B supplement.

84 Essential energy

The essential fatty acids omega-3 and omega-6 are crucial for healthy hormone function and blood sugar balance, and are needed by every cell in your body. They work to keep your skin smooth and soft, and your mood upbeat (remember that the human brain consists of more than 50 per cent fat cells). Given that fatty acids play such a vital role in health, many researchers believe that a deficiency in essential fats, especially omega-3, is a leading cause of fatigue and poor health.

To ensure you are getting your essential fats, supplement with capsules. For omega-3 this means flaxseed oil or hempseed oil capsules, or fish oil capsules. Whatever supplement you choose, read the label on the back of the container and aim for a supplement that gives you at least 150 mg of GLA (omega-6) per day. With EPA (omega-3), aim for a supplement that will give you at least 2 g per day. If you are a vegetarian and don't want to take fish oil supplements, linseed pills contain both omega-3 and omega-6 essential fats.

85 Power up with carnitine

Carnitine is a substance that can power your cells' inner engines – the mitochondria – by carrying fatty acids across cell membranes so they can be burned as energy. Foods rich in carnitine include avocados, meat and dairy products; in addition, the body makes its own supply, although this does decline with age. Studies show that 1,000 mg of carnitine daily can boost stamina and reduce fatigue, but because some forms of carnitine supplements can cause muscle weakness in high doses, if you want to give carnitine a try it is best to consult with your doctor, pharmacist or a qualified nutritionist to determine the dose that is right for you.

86 The magic of antioxidants

Antioxidants are substances found in vitamins and minerals that are crucial for your body to create energy from the food you eat. In addition to vitamin C (see page 145), vitamin E, manganese, selenium and beta carotene, which should all be included in a quality multivitamin and mineral supplement, vital energy-boosting antioxidants that you may want to supplement with include:

Alpha lipoic acid: This incredible antioxidant helps metabolise carbohydrates, proteins and fats, and keeps other energy-providing antioxidants such as vitamin C in your body for longer. You can get lipoic acid from foods like broccoli and spinach, but even if you eat lots of green leafy vegetables you are unlikely to get your recommended daily amount. Supplementing with lipoic acid can be an energy booster but, because it can lower B-vitamin stores, it is wise to consult your doctor or a nutritionist before use.

CoQ10: Co-enzyme Q10, a vitamin-like molecule present in all human tissue, is a vital catalyst for energy production because it boosts production of adenosine triphosphate (ATP), which is the molecule that fuels all your body's cells. Deficiency in this molecule can leave you feeling tired. Food sources include fish, broccoli, liver and the germ portion of wholegrains. Studies have shown that people can increase their stamina with a dose of 50–120 mg per day. To be effective, this supplement must be taken with food because it needs fat to be absorbed efficiently.

Zinc: Like vitamin C, zinc is a powerful immune-boosting vitamin that can also boost digestion and metabolism, and help balance your blood sugar. It is also crucial for mental alertness and a healthy libido. Low levels of zinc can leave you feeling tired and apathetic. Your body is more efficient at absorbing zinc from foods such as beans, pulses, fish, wholegrains, nuts and dairy foods than from tablets. Zinc is also often added to breakfast cereals; you may get your zinc this way. Much zinc gets lost in food processing, so boost your intake by eating more wholegrains, and make sure your multivitamin and mineral supplement contains zinc. If you don't think you are getting enough zinc you may want to take a daily 15-mg supplement – don't take any more than this, however, as high levels can be toxic.

87 Boost energy with herbs

A number of herbs can be added to your meals or taken as supplements to replenish your energy levels. You can buy them at the supermarket or local health food store.

Aloe Vera has been used for thousands of years as an immune-booster and skin-healer. It can also boost energy by improving digestion and blood sugar balance. Make sure that the Aloe Vera supplement you select comes with standardised extracts of Aloe Vera, otherwise it will not be as beneficial. It may cost a bit more but it will be worth it for the enhanced health benefits.

Ashwaganda is an Indian herb that seems to have potent immune-boosting and anti-stress properties. Ashwaganda has an earthy flavour that is an acquired taste, but you can also find it in most health food stores in capsule and tincture form.

Bee pollen is not strictly speaking a herb, but is often recommended by herbalists because it's one of nature's superfoods, power-packed with nutrients including amino acids, minerals, vitamins and enzymes. One or two teaspoons of fresh, raw pollen a day is suggested as an energy-booster. Some people may be allergic, so take just a few grains at first to make sure you are not.

Burdock root can be used like carrots, and boosts energy by increasing circulation.

Cinnamon is a herb widely used in cookery that can boost digestion and metabolism. Even just a little cinnamon, such as a small amount sprinkled on toast, can do the trick. A dash of cinnamon with every meal on any number of dishes may help keep blood sugar levels in check and energy levels balanced.

Garlic may have a mild blood sugar-lowering effect. And like oily fish and oats, garlic is also linked with heart health because it can lower cholesterol. Optimal doses are not known but, taking your social life into account, try to consume reasonable amounts on a regular basis. You can grate it on food, use it in cooking or take it as a one-a-day supplement in conveniently odourless capsules.

Ginger is a herb commonly used in cooking that can aid the digestive process and, in turn, increase your energy.

Gingko is great for those who tend to forget things very easily or have a hard time maintaining concentration levels. It also helps improve memory and mental alertness throughout the day.

Ginseng is a very popular product believed to help the body adapt to stress; it can help balance blood sugar levels and boost mood. Siberian ginseng – rather than the more intense Asian ginseng – is generally recommended for energy-boosting, and studies have shown that it can help combat fatigue. You can buy capsules or tinctures of Siberian ginseng at your local health food store.

Liquorice root is thought to be a powerful detoxifier that can help balance hormones. It may also have a beneficial effect on the adrenal glands, which sit on top of the kidneys and release adrenaline (the hormone that gets you up in the morning and keeps you going through the day). Liquorice is additionally known for its soothing and clearing effect on the throat, and singers often chew on it to keep their voices clear. Sweet-tasting Liquorice tea is readily available from health food stores.

Maca is marketed in some countries as an alternative to vinegar, and is known for its libido-

and stamina-boosting effects. Studies have yet to confirm this, but there is no doubt that maca is power-packed with minerals that can boost energy, such as iron and calcium.

Nettle helps balance and regulate blood sugar, which is vital for healthy energy levels. It is also mineral rich, and studies suggest that it can nourish the adrenal glands, which sit on top of the kidneys and release the get-up-and-go hormone adrenaline. You can eat nettle as a vegetable or you can make an infusion by putting 3–4 tbsp dried nettle leaves in a cup or mug of near-boiling water. Steep this for an hour, then strain. You can use the infusion as a base for soups or stews, or you can simply drink it.

Rosemary is believed to boost mental alertness and memory. To help you stay awake at your desk, put a few drops of the essential oil on a bit of cotton wool and place this on your desk.

Schisandra is a Chinese berry often used to boost mental and physical stamina. It is available at health food stores in powder or capsule form.

Spirulina is an algae and a concentrated source of high-quality, easily digestible, energy-boosting nutrients that can help balance blood sugar. It is available in tablets or in powder form.

St John's Wort has the ability to work as a mild antidepressant. Other herbs thought to boost mood include ginger, gingko, ginseng, lemon balm and peppermint.

Turmeric is a powerful herb used in curry dishes that can aid the digestive process and, in turn, increase your energy.

Stress is exhausting, and lavender, chamomile, lemon balm and passion flower are all herbs that can increase your energy by helping you relax and get more sleep. You can take any of these as a tea or a tincture any time you feel tense, or before bedtime to help you sleep. A soothing herbal bath can also aid sleep. Try adding lavender, rosemary or lemon to the water and let the soothing vapours relax and calm you.

Remember, herbs are generally safe, but caution should always be taken when you ingest them. To be on the safe side, if you are pregnant or hoping to be, are on medication or have a pre-existing medical condition like high blood pressure or diabetes, you should not use any herbs without consulting your doctor first.

Boost energy with positive thinking

88 Turn problems into puzzles

Sometimes a single word can make all the difference to your energy levels. 'Problem' is one of those words. 'Problem' is such a negative, hopeless, impotent word. When a problem descends on your life, think of it as a puzzle. Is there a way to solve this puzzle? If so, start putting the pieces together, calmly and with confidence.

'Fear' is another word that has a draining effect. Try replacing it with 'excitement' and see how different you feel. And don't stop there: turn 'failure' into 'setback', 'rejection' into 'resolution', 'obstacle' into 'opportunity'.

Once you get into the habit of rethinking your choice of words in this positive way you will notice how much easier it is to face the challenges that life throws at you.

89 Get positive

Scientists have come up with proof of the power of positive thinking. They have found that people with a sunny, optimistic outlook on life live longer, healthier and happier lives than those who are constantly worrying. The way you think has a direct influence on the way you feel and the way you behave.

If you think negative thoughts your energy levels plummet; if you think positive, upbeat thoughts, your energy levels get a boost. It is important to realise that if your thoughts are negative, you shouldn't blame yourself for the thinking patterns you have developed. They are the product of many different things over many years. But it is certainly possible to train your thoughts and develop a thinking style that is more positive.

If you are a glass-half-empty kind of person, all too often worrying and seeing the negative side becomes habitual, but an immediate change of attitude is all that it takes to turn negative thoughts into positive ones.

The next time you find yourself imagining the worst, take note of what you are doing. The first thing to change is your awareness. Then, once you realise you are being negative, just stop it. Refuse to go there and, instead, imagine the best possible outcome. Really see it happening and notice how much more energetic you feel.

The world is full of negative situations that require your attention, and positive thinking is never an excuse to bury your head in the sand. Make sure the time you spend thinking unhappy thoughts is productive: planning solutions, developing serenity or learning a valuable lesson, and remind yourself that there are just as many positive forces in the world as negative ones; your fixation on the negative is a matter of perspective and choice.

90 Sparkle with energy

Visualisation exercises in which you imagine that you are sparkling with energy and enthusiasm can be a powerful way to boost your energy and your health. This is because your mind understands images and pictures better than words, and when you imagine yourself bursting with vitality and health this provides a clear blueprint or instruction for your body and mind to put into effect.

You should practise visualisation at least once a day to maximise its energy-boosting effects. Start by sitting in a relaxed position, close your eyes and breathe deeply. Empty your mind of all thoughts and focus only on your breathing. It may take a while for your mind to clear, but when it does, imagine yourself waking up in the morning and bouncing out of bed, excited about the day ahead. See yourself glowing with energy and confidence as you move through the day and the various challenges it presents; try to use as many of your senses as possible in your energy visualisation. Don't just see; smell, taste, touch and hear what it is like to embody energy itself.

91 Say 'yes' to energy

Your mind listens to what you tell it. If you constantly tell it you are tired or run down or you can't cope, it believes you. If you tell yourself you feel energised, it will give you an instant boost. It's time to give your mind a new script. Negative self-talk lowers your energy like nothing else. Positive self-talk boosts energy, so start telling yourself that you have all the energy you need. At first it may seem strange to tell yourself that you have energy, that you can do it, that you are good enough and so on, but keep trying. You need to believe you can change for change to happen.

One tried-and-tested technique to encourage positive thinking is affirmation. Affirmations are clear statements that you consciously say to produce a desired result. They're said in the present tense to describe the positive conditions or qualities you want to experience. You state your intention to make personal transformative change. For example:

✔ I'm feeling vibrant and energetic today.
✔ I'm on top of the world.

92 Do something

A simple way to boost your energy is to switch off the TV and find something better to do. Read a book, phone a friend, write in a journal, go for a walk or learn something new. It doesn't matter what it is, as long as you enjoy it. Research shows that the feeling of having something to do is much more satisfying and stimulating than the feeling that there is nothing to do.

If you want something done, ask a busy person. Busy people tend to have more energy, more enthusiasm and are more efficient than those with less demanding schedules. This doesn't mean you should fill your day with an endless round of activity and socialising without a moment to yourself – in order to find the energy to go on, we all need downtime on a regular basis. But it does mean that you should have goals and action plans in place.

It's also important to make sure that you feel motivated. When you feel motivated about something and have a sense of purpose, it's hard to feel tired or bored – energy just seems to come naturally. Motivation, however, isn't something that always comes when you want it to. When you feel it is lacking, apply what already motivates you in other areas of your life. For example, if you never have a problem motivating yourself to play sports because you love the good feeling you get afterwards, transfer that thinking to other areas of your life where you are perhaps less motivated – doing the housework, for example. Simply think how satisfied you will feel when you get the job done.

Obviously, it isn't hard to get motivated about things that you feel passionate about or simply love to do; so, whether your passion is dancing, singing, reading, crosswords or fly fishing, try to make time for it. If you can't think of anything you are passionate about, ask yourself what you would do if you had all the money in the world and no constraints on your time.

On those days when you feel really low in energy and that your life is missing something, find a new sense of purpose by offering to help someone less fortunate than you. Visit your local volunteer centre and offer your skills and time. Giving to others will add meaning, purpose and energy to your own life.

93 Become a motivator

Who do you know who needs some encouragement, inspiration or motivation to boost their energy and performance? Perhaps it's a colleague or your partner or a child. Perhaps it's you. One of the most successful ways to give yourself a positive energy boost is to inspire or encourage someone else.

So how do you become a motivator? Easy! Think of someone who encouraged you. What did they say? What did they do? If you can't think of anyone, imagine what could get you motivated. What could someone say to you? How could someone help you to succeed? Now look around and find someone who needs some encouragement, or someone who seems a little short on self-belief. Low self-esteem is one of the most de-energising forces of them all. It doesn't just zap confidence. It zaps energy and enthusiasm, too. Encourage them to be the best that they can be and to do what they can rather than focusing on what they can't do. Remind them of how special and unique they are, and tell them that they deserve the very best.

94 Less is more

Perfectionist beliefs are another key factor that increases stress and drains energy. Perfectionists can never win in life since nothing in their lives is ever perfect. There is always something, however small, that can be improved. This means a perfectionist is always falling short of the unrealistic standards they set themselves and can never appreciate what they have achieved.

A perfectionist fails to recognise what is known as the '80/20 rule'. This means that if you can get things 80 per cent right you are doing really well and have high standards – any more than that is a real bonus. Very few things in real life ever add up to 100 per cent.

This is not to say you should not want or expect the best from life. It is simply saying that absolute perfection is an impossible ideal that can drain rather than motivate.

95 Show your teeth

Humour has the power to break us out of our rut, to make us see things in a new light and to boost our energy. So try to laugh and play as much as you can, as laughter and playtime are guaranteed to put a spring in your step and more light in your eyes.

If you smile, you'll notice several things: smiles are contagious, and they actually boost your energy and improve your mood. People respond to smiles with friendliness and generosity, which could turn your whole day around. Smiles even work when you are chatting on the telephone, as they can be recognised clearly by the person on the other end.

If you don't feel like smiling, imagine yourself laughing, and then trying not to laugh as if you were in a church or library. This exercise will soon have the corners of your mouth lifted and, while you are smiling, squeeze your thumb and forefinger together to create a mental anchor you can repeat later in the day to take you back to that energetic moment.

96 Reach out

Every day, life presents you with another opportunity to say something kind, generous and genuine to somebody. Whether it's complimenting a co-worker on his new tie, admiring someone's accomplishment or telling a loved one you care, boosting the positive energy in someone else's life boosts it in your own, too.

A 10-year Australian study has shown that positive relationships with others and the support of good friends and family are associated with how long we live, how healthy we stay and how good we feel about ourselves. It's hard to feel negative and tired when you are surrounded by people who love and understand you, so nourish and cherish those people you care about.

Do make sure that the people with whom you surround yourself are positive and supportive. There is nothing more energy-draining than people who complain, criticise or undermine all the time. Avoid people like that, or at least try to minimise your contact with them.

97 An attitude of gratitude

Being thankful for what is good in your life can make all the difference to your energy levels. In fact, there is a growing movement among psychologists, called 'positive psychology', which actively promotes the power of optimism. So, instead of seeing your glass as half-empty, try to see it as half-full; find the good rather than the bad in situations and people, and feel grateful rather than burdened down by your responsibilities. Start viewing your daily routine as a privilege, not as a chore.

The human tendency is always to want more or to think the grass is greener on the other side of the fence, but a better approach is to remember where you began and how much you have already accomplished. The more grateful you are for the gift of your life, the more positive your life will become and the more energy you will have to live it to the full.

Boost mental energy

98 Break your routine

If your mind stagnates, your energy does, too. So be as open to new experiences as possible, be they painting or paragliding, sailing or singing. We spend so much of our day going through tried-and-tested routines, with our minds and eyes blinkered, that we forget to open our mind and our eyes. Next time you are on the bus, train or in a taxi, look out of the window, then look away and try to recall all the new things that you hadn't noticed before.

Keep stimulating your mind by chopping and changing the ingredients in your life; as you spice up the ingredients, your morning leap will follow suit. Learn something new, listen to music or read books that you normally wouldn't, change your holiday destination to somewhere you've never been before. Find ways to add as much spice and variety into your life as possible; your brain will love it.

99 Do the cross-over

The left hemisphere of your brain controls the right side of your body and vice versa. In most people the left side of the brain is the logical side. It deals with facts, dates, letters, maths skills and language. Timing and rhythm, necessary for music skills, are here, too. The right side deals with colour, imagery, perspective and spatial awareness. Imagination, intuition and insight are located here, along with the ability to recognise and remember tones and sounds. Put simply, the right brain recognizes faces and the left brain recognises names, and it's only when both sides of your brain are engaged that you can reach your full learning potential.

Anything that can stimulate both sides of your brain will boost your mental energy and powers of concentration, so try writing, brushing your teeth or combing your hair with your non-dominant hand. As you walk, swing your hand across your body towards the opposite leg. Learn to play the piano or another musical instrument that is easier for beginners, such as the recorder or drums. Pat your stomach with your right hand and make an imaginary circle above your head with your left hand. Now swap hands. Keep practising until it is easy on both sides and you will have successfully 'crossed your wires'.

These cross-over exercises will boost your alertness whatever age you are. Contrary to popular belief, your brain power does not decline with old age. It can repair itself and create new pathways of thought and memory. Every time you stimulate your brain, a unique network of connections is activated. If you have acquired a new skill or learned something new, this creates yet more connections, as well as strengthening the ones you already have.

The more you use your brain the better it gets. It's a case of 'use it or lose it', so find ways to sharpen your reflexes and enhance your mental energy. Learn a new language or do crosswords, puzzles, word games and card games. Bridge and sudoku help promote spatial orientation and boost concentration and creativity. Encourage your own mental challenges, and let your brain and your energy grow.

100 Buy a yo-yo!

Toys can boost your mental energy by boosting your concentration, improving your hand–eye coordination and engaging your creativity; so treat yourself to a new toy. Buy some Lego to build a motorbike or a cruise ship, get a yo-yo or some battery-operated cars, and see how quick your reflexes are. Toys are made for children to have fun with, using their minds and imagination at the same time; they can have a similar effect on adults.

If the thought of toys doesn't appeal, you can get three tennis balls and have a go at juggling. Studies show that learning to juggle can increase your brain power because it requires focus, rhythm and coordination, and can improve your motor skills and spatial awareness. It's also fun and a great way to take your mind off the worries and stresses that drain your energy. If you have never juggled before or it has been a while since you used a yo-yo or built a Lego house, expect to feel clumsy and uncoordinated at first. If you keep practising you will soon notice your creativity and mental energy return.

PART THREE:

INSTANT PICK-ME-UPS: RECHARGE IN 60 SECONDS OR LESS

Pop a peppermint

The strong aroma of peppermint wakes you up, much like smelling salts. The mint scent stimulates a nerve in your brain, making you feel more alert. Sucking or chewing mints delivers an even bigger energy kick than just smelling it. When you eat these aromatic sweets, odour molecules circulating in your mouth drift up your nose via the back of your throat, multiplying the scent's intensity. Pop a mint any time you're feeling low, or chew some peppermint gum for a minute or two. Studies show that chewing peppermint gum stimulates the same part of the brain that wakes you up in the morning.

The power behind bananas

If you want a quick fix for flagging energy levels, there is no better snack than a banana. Containing three natural sugars – sucrose, fructose and glucose – combined with fibre, a banana gives an instant, sustained and substantial boost of energy. Research has shown that just two bananas provide enough energy for a strenuous 90-minute workout. No wonder the banana is the number-one fruit with the world's leading athletes.

Get an ATP fix

Your body needs a good supply of ATP, which is the molecule that supplies energy to all your cells. It is found in vegetables and wholegrains, but one of the best sources is pumpkin seeds. Studies show that when women had 50 g a day as mid-meal snacks, 80 per cent reported having more energy.

Spritz yourself

Carry a spray bottle of water around with you. If your energy dips, a light spritz on your face will revive you.

Pump up the volume

When your energy sags during the day or night, put on some music with a dance or up-tempo beat. Music, in particular Mozart, has been shown by many studies to help boost mood and alertness, and add a little sparkle to our lives.

Tarzan power

A few inches down from your collar bone and just above your heart is your thymus gland, which is important for the healthy functioning of your immune system. Some energy practitioners encourage tapping the thymus gland to stimulate energy.

Try a boron boost

Research has shown that people with enough boron in their diet are more alert and can concentrate better than those who are deficient. Raisins are a good source of boron and energy-boosting iron, so you kill two birds with one stone when you carry a small packet of raisins around with you.

Rest your forehead

Place your elbow on the table and rest your forehead on the heel of your palm, or simply hold your fingertips to your forehead. According to energy practitioners, touching the neuro-vascular points on your forehead keeps blood circulating to your forebrain and revitalises you.

Hum

Singing is a natural energy-booster that can lift your mood, ease stress and put you in harmony with your surroundings. Research also shows that people who sing have healthier lungs and fitness levels than those who don't. It doesn't matter how good your voice is, just open your mouth, take a breath and let the sounds come out. Sing in the shower, at home or wherever you can. If it isn't possible to sing, simply hum. When you hum, feel the vibrations enliven your senses, stimulate your mind and expand your chest.

Yawn

Scientists still don't know why we yawn, but it is possible that we yawn to re-energise ourselves by increasing oxygen consumption. If your energy dips – and you aren't in the middle of an important discussion or meeting – try making yourself yawn to see if it helps.

Rub your ears

Stimulating certain pressure points on your body increases your blood circulation – and thus your energy – according to proponents of Traditional Chinese Medicine. Using your fingers, vigorously rub your ears all over for about 1 minute. (Don't be so rough that you hurt yourself, but do expect your ears to feel hot, a sign that your blood is circulating.) Almost immediately, you should feel more alert.

Take a power shower

To shake off morning grogginess, stand under steaming hot water and rub your entire body with a washcloth, preferably with eucalyptus-, peppermint- or citrus-scented soap, as these scents can stimulate your brain. The hot water and the rubdown speed blood flow, sending oxygen to your cells where it's transformed into energy. Finish up your shower with a blast of cool or cold water. The temperature change instantly triggers your nervous system's fight-or-flight response, which will make you feel wide awake.

Give your eyes a wash

If your eyes feel tired it can be hard to feel energetic and upbeat, so buy some eye drops and, the next time you feel the strain, give your eyes a refreshing wash.

Wear sunglasses

Reflected harsh light can strain your eyes, causing headaches and fatigue. To adjust to the glare, use sunglasses when you are outside; if you are indoors, move your seat, close the blinds or add softer light.

Try a cold rub

Dip a washcloth or small towel in cold water and wrap it around your hand or face for an invigorating lift.

Sniff a pine cone

There is an aromatic oil in fir, pine and spruce cones that stimulates the nose to release adrenaline, and this can give you an instant boost.

Shrug it off

If your shoulders are rigid, the flow of blood and oxygen to the brain becomes obstructed. Relax your shoulders and give yourself an instant

energy boost by pulling your shoulders up to
your ears, holding for a count of 10 and then
dropping them as you exhale with a sigh.

Refocus your eyes

If your eyes are tired, you are more likely to feel
tired. Flexible eyes work better than fixated ones,
so a simple energiser is to remember to look into
the distance out of a window or to the end of the
room at a picture every 20 minutes or so if you
are reading or working on a computer. You could
also hold your finger close to your nose and then
look beyond your finger to a point in the
distance. Do this 5 times.

Drink cold water

This wakes up the sedentary muscles and gets
them moving again. An added benefit: drinking
cold water increases fat-burning potential as it
requires more calories and energy to get that
water to body temperature. Even better, add
some fruit juice to your cold water and ice to
give your body a nourishing energy shot.

Let the light in

Open the windows and curtains, lift the shades and let some energising fresh air in. And if you've got time, take a stroll in the sunlight to increase your natural antidepressants. Dopamine, endorphins and other chemicals in the brain kick into high gear with the combination of sunlight and motion. The effect can last for up to 5 hours.

Ergonomics 101

Sitting all day in front of a computer can be an enormous strain on your eyes, so make sure your feet are flat on the floor when you sit down, your back is straight and your head level with the monitor. Your elbows should bend at 90° with your hands comfortable on the keyboard. If you are typing from a book or piece of paper, prop it up so you don't have to bend your head to read.

Choose the power seat

If you find it hard to stay alert in meetings, take what is called the 'power seat' facing the door.

Seeing who is coming in or out helps you stay more energised. In a class or presentation, sit next to the teacher or speaker.

Rub your hands

Put the palms of your hands together and rub them vigorously for 1 minute, imagining that stress is leaving your body through your fingertips. Afterwards you'll feel more motivated.

Visualise energy

Breathe deeply and imagine a yellow and orange band of energy flowing around your body for 1 minute.

Blossom

A bunch of flowers is one of the simplest and easiest ways to feel better instantly. The beauty, colour and scent of flowers are stimulating, which is why they always appear in depictions of paradise.

Change your light bulbs

If you can't work near a window or outside, a full-spectrum light bulb or a fluorescent light provide more light than standard light bulbs. Try a full-spectrum light in your office or sitting room; you may find it boosts your energy because it will be easier for your eyes to focus.

Put your shoes on and take them off

If you work from home, you may find that you feel more capable, accomplished and energetic if you work with your shoes on. However, when you have finished your work or get home after a busy day, take your shoes off and wear slippers or go barefoot instead. This will give you an instant energy release.

Brush your teeth

An instant way to revive you and make it feel like morning again is to brush your teeth with peppermint or spearmint toothpaste.

Stand on your head

Studies have shown that turning yourself upside-down can boost memory and alertness. It reverses the usual pull of gravity, boosts circulation and gives a sense of renewal. If you can't stand on your head, sit down on a chair and put your head between your knees. Stay there for a minute before slowly returning to an upright position.

Scratch your head

This is something you probably do without thinking about it when you want to come up with a solution to a problem. What you may not know is that scratching can help the blood flow to the brain. To get the full benefits, scratch lightly with your fingertips, not your nails. Start at the base of your skull where your spine meets your head, as this will stimulate the spinal nerves that connect to your brain. Then scratch each temple and work in an arc shape around your ears. Alternatively, you could just run your fingertips all over your skull.

Sniff a lemon

When you find your energy dipping, sniff a ripe lemon as the scent of citrus fruits can increase alertness. According to the Smell and Taste Treatment Research Foundation, other energy-boosting scents include orange, lime, grapefruit, rosemary, ginger, eucalyptus, spearmint and peppermint.

See red

Stare at something red. The colour is an instant pick-me-up, as it energises and increases adrenaline production, heart rate and blood pressure. Though red flowers are ideal for their 'red' power, their scent and the sentiment attached to them, anything red will do: a handbag, a sweater or even a piece of red paper.

Light up your morning

Research has shown that if you put your bedside light on a timer to turn on half an hour before you wake up, you will feel more energetic in the morning. It may not work for everyone, but try it and find out.

Liven up your desktop

If you spend long hours on the computer each day, changing the colours or pictures in your computing environment will help reinvigorate your desk time. Your brain gets used to images fairly quickly, so to keep it stimulated change your screen set-up every few days.

Skip

This is an instant pick-me-up that you can do anywhere. If you feel fatigue setting in, get up and skip around the room for 1 minute, like a child in the playground. Your blood circulation and your mood will get an instant boost.

Make it a latte

As long as you don't drink more than two cups a day, it's fine to enjoy a stimulating cup of coffee when you feel your concentration and energy dipping. A protein-rich milky latte will boost your stamina as well as your concentration. Try to avoid drinking coffee after 3 p.m., though, as it takes a while for caffeine to leave your system and this could stop you getting a good night's sleep.

And finally ... breathe out

Breathing in deeply is often recommended to help boost energy, but it is also important to breathe out deeply to get rid of old stagnant air before you take in a breath of revitalizing oxygen. When we breathe normally we get rid of only about 20 per cent of the air in our lungs, so when your energy is low take a deep breath in and then breathe out for a few moments longer than you normally would. Exhaling deeply will naturally make your next intake of breath deeper. You will immediately feel yourself becoming more alert with every breath. And when you feel more alert, your energy levels increase instantly and you can enjoy the present moment and your life as a whole as it should always be enjoyed – to the full.

INDEX